Advancing Quality

Total Quality Management in
the National Health Service

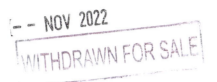

Service

Health Services Management

Series Editors:
Chris Ham, Health Services Management Centre, University of Birmingham
Chris Heginbotham, The Riverside Mental Health Trust, London

The British National Health Service is one of the biggest and most complex organizations in the developed world. Employing around one million people and accounting for £36 billion of public expenditure, the service is of major concern to both the public and politicians. Management within the NHS faces a series of challenges in ensuring that resources are deployed efficiently and effectively. These challenges include the planning and management of human resources, the integration of professionals into the management process, and making sure that services meet the needs of patients and the public.

Against this background, the Health Services Management series addresses the many issues and practical problems faced by people in managerial roles in health services.

Current and forthcoming titles

Advancing Quality

Total Quality Management in the National Health Service

Richard Joss and Maurice Kogan

Open University Press
Buckingham · Philadelphia

Open University Press
Celtic Court
22 Ballmoor
Buckingham
MK18 1XW

and

1900 Frost Road, Suite 101
Bristol, PA 19007, USA

First Published 1995

A catalogue record of this book is available from the British Library

ISBN   0 335 19395 1 (pb)   0 335 19396 X (hb)

Library of Congress Cataloging-in-Publication Data
Joss, Richard, 1945–
  Advancing quality: Total quality management in the National Health Service/
  Richard Joss and Maurice Kogan.
      p.   cm. — (Health services management)
    Includes bibliographical references and index.
    ISBN 0–335–19395–1 (pbk.). — ISBN 0–335–19396–X (hb)
    1. Medical care—Great Britain—Quality control. 2. National Health
Service (Great Britain) 3. Total quality management. 4. National Health
Service (Great Britain) I. Kogan, Maurice. II. Title. III. Series.
    [DNLM: 1. Total Quality Management—methods. 2. State Medicine—
organization & administration. 3. State Medicine—organization &
administration—Great Britain. W 275 J97t FA1   1995]
RA399.G7J67   1995
362.1'0941—dc20
DNLM/DLC
for Library of Congress   95–15493
                                                                                  CIP

Typeset by Graphicraft Ltd, Hong Kong
Printed in Great Britain by Biddles Ltd, Guildford and King's Lynn

Contents

Preface

This book will be helpful to the large numbers of people working in the National Health Service who are concerned to improve quality. It explains the many different meanings of quality as they can be applied to the delivery of health care, and suggests ways in which professionals, managers and those working at the operational levels can identify quality problems and do something about them.

In producing this work we are left in debt to many colleagues in the field. In particular, we are grateful to our Brunel colleague, Mary Henkel, who shared the fieldwork and analysis involved in our study. The Department of Health invited us to evaluate their Total Quality Management experiment which was an ambitious attempt to promote and test changes in attitudes and working in the NHS. Without their sponsorship we could not have entered this field of work.

Our evaluation involved us in nearly 750 one-hour interviews with staff at 38 different hospitals and community service units and 12 health authorities over three years. We also carried out over 100 interviews with staff at 12 locations in two commercial companies, Post Office Counters and Thames Water, during the same period. This work could not have been undertaken without wholehearted cooperation from those with whom we worked. We cannot name them all, but we are deeply grateful to them.

At the conclusion of our report we submitted a substantial technical report to the Department of Health which remains available to our fellow researchers and others who might want to examine the basis upon which some of our conclusions rest. This book is, however, intended for those who wish to take effective action through quality initiatives.

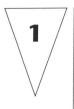

1 What this book is about

Embarking on Total Quality Management (TQM) in any organization, least of all the NHS, is not a decision to be taken lightly. TQM requires a wholehearted and long-term commitment to a particular approach to quality improvement. It has its origins in private sector manufacturing and has only relatively recently made a somewhat uneasy transition to service industries. The cultural, structural and systems differences between private sector services and public sector health suggest that considerable thought needs to be given to how the principles of TQM could be operationalized in the NHS.

One of the major concerns would be how to define quality, given the different perceptions and requirements of different groups of staff and the wide range of stakeholders in the NHS – government, regional and district purchasers, trust boards, doctors, paramedics, nurses, patients, clients and their carers, to name just some of the interested parties. In the past, most definitions of quality of health care would have focused on technical and professional definitions. However, over the last 15 years in the USA, and more recently in Britain, there has been a move towards consumer-oriented definitions of quality in service delivery.

Our model of quality (expanded upon in Chapter 8) puts forward a concept of quality which has three dimensions or modes – what we have called *technical, systemic* and *generic* quality. *Technical* quality is concerned with the technical-professional content of work within a given area; *systemic* quality refers to the quality of systems and processes that operate across the boundaries between areas of work; and *generic* quality refers to those aspects of quality which involve inter-personal relationships including standards of civility, punctuality and respect for the worth of others.

A day in the life of an outpatients' department

The three modes of quality can best be described by way of an example. Consider the following case, which is drawn from our evaluation of TQM in the NHS. There are three players, each of whom is grappling with a complex issue of quality. First, a consultant in an outpatients' clinic who is considering the results from a medical audit study of the effectiveness of a particular diagnostic procedure. This procedure has been the standard approach for many years but is gradually giving way to the use of a new piece of equipment which might make the old technique redundant. For some months now she has been running both procedures in parallel but the time has come to decide whether or not to continue with the new equipment on its own.

The doctor sees her problem as primarily one of *technical* quality. Of course, in the back of her mind she is also aware of the resource implications of each procedure (which may lead to *systemic* problems) just as she is concerned about the dignity of patients subjected to the procedure (*generic* quality). However, the procedure is used to identify a life-threatening condition, and she cannot afford to change to a new test which might fail to detect vital signs – hence her preoccupation with technical issues.

Meanwhile, the supplies manager is grappling with his own concerns. These reflect the need to be able to supply all his internal customers (including outpatients) with anything they might require at a moment's notice but at the same time keep inventory as low as possible. This is important for two reasons: first, he is running out of space in the stores; and second, he wants to keep as little cash tied up in goods as possible.

The supplies manager wants to keep his promises to his customers (*generic* quality) and is aware of issues surrounding the storage life of certain medical products (*technical* quality), but he sees his problem as mainly one of logistics because he has to supply many different departments, each of which has its own requirements, systems and procedures (*systemic* quality). It is the systemic issues which he will often see as the major determinants of quality.

The third player in this little drama is the outpatients manager. She is trying to sort out some complaints from patients. Two complaints are uppermost in her mind at the moment – the heat in the waiting areas (too hot for some patients and too cold for others), and the attitudes of some staff who she feels 'seem to think the hospital runs for their benefit rather than that of the patients'.

In our example, the outpatients manager is primarily concerned to meet her patients' needs about their immediate comfort and the way they are treated by others (*generic* quality). She realizes that problems with the central heating are to do with whether or not it is the right equipment for the job, and how it is serviced and operated (*technical* quality). She is also aware that the matter of staff attitudes is underpinned by broader issues of recruitment, selection, training and reward which go well beyond the boundaries of the outpatients' department (*systemic* quality). However, her personal concerns have always been focused on the individual needs of her patients. With the increased attention to patient measures of satisfaction she finds more and more of her time is now spent on generic issues.

If the concerns of these three staff were not complicated enough, consider what happens when the doctor decides to go over to the new procedure. Because her interest is mainly in *technical* quality, she forgets to tell the other two managers. The first the supplies manager knows about the decision is when the materials he used to supply for the old procedure begin to pile up, throwing out his storage systems. Also, because they have a limited shelf-life, some have to be discarded and an appreciable amount of money is wasted.

Meanwhile, the outpatients manager finds that the new procedure changes the flow of patients through the clinic, causing a rash of new complaints from some patients but pleasing those having the new procedure. Staff, who were not prepared for the changes, also complain about lack of consideration and training. They demand to be upgraded because the new procedure is more complex. Financial estimates made in the budget now look threatened. At the next meeting of the Management Committee the Chief Executive announces that everyone will shortly be required to introduce a new initiative called Total Quality Management. No one should be concerned 'because TQM has been very successful in improving quality in Japanese car plants . . .'!

What is to be done about quality in the NHS?

How, then, should we go about improving the quality of public sector health care services? What have quality assurance (QA) and TQM got to offer the NHS and how can they be modified to meet the particular requirements of the NHS's competing stakeholders?

We have set out to answer these questions in three stages. First, we review the theoretical and conceptual issues surrounding models of quality improvement. Then we report our extensive evaluation of TQM in the NHS which also took in TQM programmes in the commercial sector. Finally, we consider the options for improving on QA in the NHS and put forward our own model as part of an agenda for reform.

We have tried to cover as many of the practical considerations of designing and evaluating a QA programme as possible. However, we are also concerned that much of the latest quality improvement activity in the NHS, particularly that which follows TQM approaches, is not well thought out and has little regard for some of the key literature on organizational development. We therefore consider it important to provide a critique of existing models of TQM rather than just an elaboration of them.

The plan of the book

Chapter 2 asks 'what is quality?' and goes on to consider ways to improve it – matters that are taken up again in Chapter 8. It shows how

TQM has developed from commercial approaches to quality improvement and how it is being adapted from use in the private sector into a model of quality assurance for the NHS.

In Chapter 3 we take up methods of designing for quality. Much writing on quality takes little account of work undertaken on organizational change. We note which models of change might be thought to be most appropriate for quality implementation and ways of designing this implementation within the NHS.

Chapter 4 takes up a matter which causes some uncertainty within the NHS, namely, how quality initiatives might be evaluated. We look at some of the measures which are available for evaluating the extent to which quality has improved and also consider ways of evaluating full projects for installing TQM.

Chapter 5 describes some of the lessons to be derived from our work in the 38 different NHS service units over our three-year evaluation.

Chapter 6 considers what can be learned from the commercial sector, particularly as viewed from our study of quality implementation in Post Office Counters and Thames Water. As well as considering what might be learned, we analyse why commercial quality practices might not work in the NHS.

Chapter 7 draws together the significance of what we have found in both the NHS and commercial organizations, and Chapter 8 provides an agenda for reform in terms of both more orthodox forms of TQM and through our new model of QA for the NHS.

The appendices should be useful to those wanting to follow up particular methods of implementation or evaluation. We have also provided a bibliography of some of the more accessible writing on quality and quality improvement.

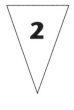

2 What do we mean by quality and quality improvement?

Introduction

The quest for quality is made the more testing by the difficulty of defining it. While the drive for quality improvement is as strong in the National Health Service (NHS) as in any other public or private sector organization, it would be a mistake to assume that it is underpinned by common understandings of quality either within the NHS or between the NHS and other organizations. Within the NHS definitions of quality vary profoundly between different groups of staff and between staff and patients. We will be looking at this issue in some detail, both in this chapter and later in Chapter 5.

First, though, we examine the more general changes in ideas about quality that have occurred throughout Western society since the 1930s. Today, 'Working for Quality' would typically be the slogan of a Total Quality Management (TQM) company. However, before the Second World War, it would almost certainly have been a phrase used by working-class domestic staff to refer to the status of their employers. As Pfeffer and Coote (1991, p. 4) note, this early concept of quality was based on traditional notions of exclusivity, prestige and positional advantage. The authors go on to discuss several substantial changes since that time and argue for a shift towards what they call a democratic approach (see Table 2.1).

The changes that Pfeffer and Coote discuss have been shaped by social, political, technical and organizational developments. These have combined in complex ways which defy detailed causal analysis. However, general trends can be observed and it is important to be aware of these when analysing current perceptions of quality in the 'new-style' NHS. Figure 2.1 charts some of the developments which have framed the context for the changes described by Pfeffer and Coote.

Table 2.1   Changing concepts of quality

General approach	Key features and issues
Traditional approach	Quality is conceived as exclusiveness, prestige and positional advantage; by definition, most people would not have access to this quality.
Expert approach	Specifications of a product or service are defined by scientists and other experts or professionals; quality is linked to fitness for purpose; there is a rational and analytic evaluation of outcomes, but professional viewpoints are narrow and participation by users is lacking.
Managerial/excellence approach	Quality is defined by customer satisfaction in a competitive environment; hierarchical organizations are flattened and staff empowered to be more responsive to customer needs; customers may express satisfaction with existing services but may be unaware of alternatives – they are mainly passive participants in the process of service definition; tests of opinion are mostly *post hoc*.
Consumerist approach	Active participation by customers in shaping services through their purchasing behaviour; the issues here are 'exit v. voice' (Hirschman, 1970); there is little by way of a role for non-consumers; the complex roles of people as citizens are ignored. This approach tends to increase power of exit rather than giving people a voice. In the NHS context it may also push less efficient/effective providers into a spiral of decline rather than improve performance.
Democratic approach	Need for equality based on fitness for purpose (expert/ scientific), responsiveness (excellence), empowerment (consumerist), plus involvement of staff, public participation (whether consumers or not), enforceable rights, open management.

Source: Adapted from Pfeffer and Coote (1991).

In most cases the general trend in the public sector has been one of a move from definitions of quality (held by professional, technical or political groups) that are either narrow and technical or vague and intuitive, towards definitions based on a complex mixture of stakeholders' views. This move has led to a search for more holistic models that might allow for multiple perceptions of needs and wants. In the case of the NHS, the driving force included technical and financial concerns about the rising costs of providing advanced medical care to an increasingly ageing population. One approach, among many adopted by Conservative governments,

Figure 2.1 General trends in the development of concepts of quality in the public and private sectors

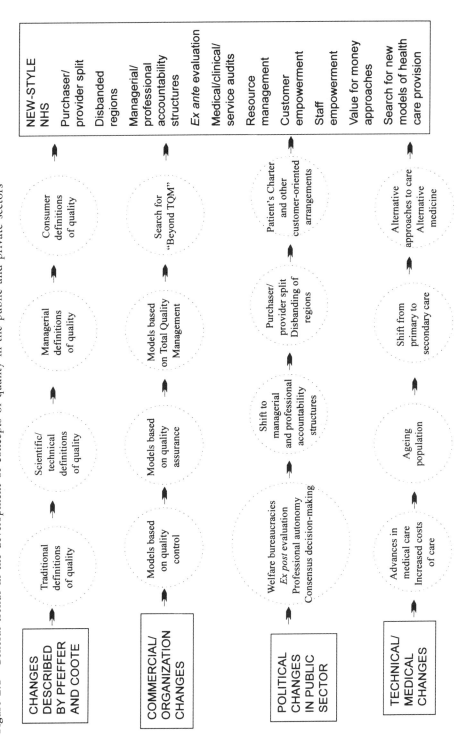

Table 2.2 A comparison of changes being made in the NHS and some of the basic principles of TQM

NHS changes	*TQM principles*
Strengthening top management at each unit and involving doctors in management of services	Corporate approaches to planning, especially planning for quality – working towards common understandings and definitions
Value for money	Continuous improvement through systematic measurement
Greater patient focus, including more information, more choice and more involvement	Putting the customer at the centre of process improvement

was to push through reforms designed to focus on providing value for money through increased efficiency and wider consumer choice. Models of TQM in the private sector, where the stress was also on customer-driven quality improvement, seemed a natural addition to that change process. Table 2.2 shows how the principles of TQM could be seen to correspond to the NHS changes.

Commercial approaches to quality improvement

We begin our review of approaches to quality improvement with the manufacturing sector, where much of the early work started. We track developments from the early days of quality control (QC), through QA, to its present-day conception as TQM. We then contrast these manufacturing process models with more recent work on service quality and explore the extent to which other major quality initiatives such as medical audit, British Standards 5750, and standard setting are in keeping with the models of TQM now being implemented in the NHS. The analysis in this chapter provides the background to the development of criteria which we suggest may be used to evaluate TQM in the NHS (Chapter 3).

The influence of industrialization on quality

Concerns with quality in the manufacturing sector have been expressed since goods were first made and services delivered. However, the responses to problems of poor quality in manufacturing have shifted dramatically in the last hundred years or so. These shifts may be seen as responses to changes in production processes brought about by: industrialization; increased specialization; automation and computerization; increased complexity of production (with a consequent rise in the proportion of bought-in components); and the application of scientific methods of management. One of the results of these shifts was a decline in the number of skilled workers who were responsible for a complete production process and an increase in employment of unskilled and semi-skilled workers carrying out high-volume repetitive sub-tasks in narrow areas of production.

The sense of individual ownership of quality for the final product proved difficult to maintain under these conditions and an early response was the introduction of formal QC systems. These may be traced back to the early 1920s with the use of control charts and statistical process control by Shewhart at Bell Telephone Laboratories (Shewhart, 1931). QC was an attempt to move from inspection processes that were designed to identify and remove faulty products during production, to controls aimed at increasing the percentage of good products being manufactured. The Shewhart problem-solving cycle, *Plan–Do–Check–Act*, still forms the basis of most QC and QA systems today (Neave, 1990).

A typical commercial sector example is the approach used in Post Office Counters' successful TQM initiative (See Chapter 6 and Figure 2.2). First one prioritizes the areas for improvement and then selects a specific area. The next stage *(focus)* emphasizes the importance of the customer since one must first identify the gap between current outputs and the customer requirements. The causes of the gap are analysed and potential solutions are designed to reduce the gap *(plan)*. Implementation of the chosen solution *(do)* is followed by systematic monitoring and evaluation *(review)* before going round the cycle again.

As Crosby (1979) has argued, a whole culture developed during the post-war years in which manufacturers accepted the inevitability of errors occurring in production. It was quite common for producers to allow a certain percentage of defective goods to go out to customers. The exact percentage was viewed as a trade-off between costs of assuring perfection, and levels of customer dissatisfaction. Indeed, the practice was known well enough for it to have its own acronym – AQL (acceptable quality levels). Reworking rejected products became a way of life, with a consequent rise in related cost areas such as inventory.

From quality control to quality assurance

After the Second World War, the emphasis changed from quality control to quality assurance. The result was increased attention to pre-production planning where everything possible was done systematically to design out errors in production processes. It became clear that most errors could be attributed to process design. In fact, we now see the development of a whole new science of statistical methods for *off-line* quality management (see, for example, Kackar, 1985).

The 'quality revolution', however, is held to have taken place in Japan from the early 1950s onwards. The people credited with driving this revolution were Deming and Juran (Macdonald and Piggott, 1990). Deming's approach proved particularly attractive to the Japanese. His early work depended to a large extent on identifying the causes of variation in

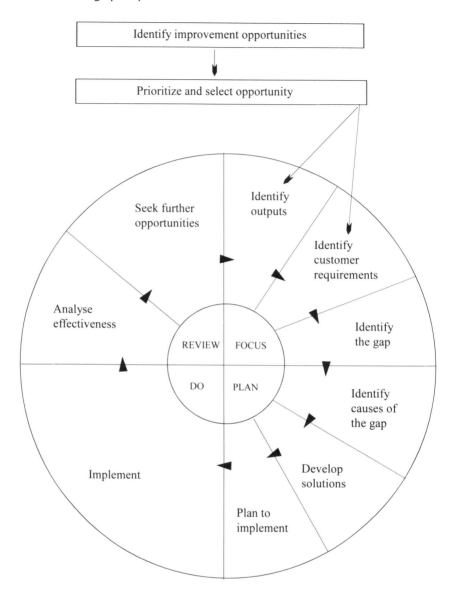

Figure 2.2   Post Office Counters' quality improvement process

production processes and where possible systematically reducing it through the use of a range of statistical tools. He later went on to propose methods for the development of a quality culture through motivating and developing people (see, for example, Deming, 1986).

The early statistical processes, based on detection, were broadened to encompass prevention. It is important to note, too, that this shift to QA (first tested in Japan by Deming and Juran) contained appreciable elements of worker empowerment, since the workers were expected to contribute to identifying causes of variation, and planning basic changes in working practice.

From quality assurance to Total Quality Management

As QA widened in scope, it became clear that there were severe limitations in the extent to which any group of workers could influence change. The first limitation was that the early problem-solving teams were mainly intra-departmental and often uni-disciplinary. Since production processes spanned inter-departmental boundaries, production workers found that they had little influence on engineering, materials, personnel and so on. Second, it was found that the overwhelming majority of significant improvements required changes in policy or cross-functional practice that were the province of managers (see, for example, Macdonald and Piggott, 1990).

The result was a broadening of QA to take in all activities within an organization and, more recently, to extend the process of QA to the organization's external suppliers. Structured quality improvement initiatives, which began with shop-floor production processes, were also extended to the upper reaches of organizations, and programmes became increasingly corporate and top-down in outlook. Quality statements began to appear in company mission statements and quality plans featured as part of the normal business planning process.

The rise in consumerism

Paralleling these developments were changes in perceptions about the importance of the consumer. Until the 1950s, definitions of quality tended to revolve around what experts thought the customer wanted, or should or could have. Within companies, major decisions about new products were made on the advice of experts in research and development departments or marketing specialists. Quality standards were defined by experts in costing, by production technologists and by guidance from national standard-setting bodies such as the British Standards Institution.

With the rise in consumerism, particularly in the USA, and the famous safety 'debates' between Ralph Nader and major car manufacturers (Nader, 1965), attention switched to how far consumers had a voice in product specification and development. Several consumer organizations were established in Britain, most notably the Consumers' Association in 1957 and the National Consumers' Council in 1975. Consumer groups began to badger companies for more information about their products, and the practice of carrying out comparative tests of products from different producers became more common.

This pressure led to increasing competition in the market place. There was a boom in market surveys as companies rushed to find out what their customers wanted. In order better to track and respond to changes in consumer demand, many organizations were urged to restructure in order to push accountability 'down the line', reduce the number of hierarchical levels, and empower front-line staff by involving them in decision-making (see, for example, Peters, 1989). Quality became everyone's business and the driving force was to meet (and, if possible, exceed) customer requirements in as cost-effective way as possible. But this focus on customers did little in reality to empower them. Customers could, for example, express satisfaction with a product because they were not told about its less desirable features, or because they were not aware of better alternatives. In so far as the consumers could exercise choice, it was their purchasing power which provided the real check.

When we turn to the welfare services, however, the issues revolve around the extent to which consumers can affect the design and delivery of care in the absence of the checks offered by economic choice. While public sector clients may be empowered by increasing the opportunities for them to have a voice, they have hitherto had no power of exit (Hirschman, 1970). Indeed exercising the exit option may profit individuals as consumers but may be harmful if one takes into account their wider role as people who also have a stake in the service as citizens and members of the wider community. For example, where a service is over-subscribed, the providers might be grateful for 'one less in the queue', as it were – in this case, exercising the option of exit has unintended effects (see Pfeffer and Coote, 1991, who argue that voice may be more important than exit).

What, then, is TQM?

TQM has its origins in private sector manufacturing and its importation, first to the commercial services sector, and then to the public sector, is a relatively recent phenomenon. Indeed, it was more or less unheard of in the public sector in Britain until about the mid-1980s. Its importation has not been without problems and modifications have had to be made to the way it is implemented, if not to some of the assumptions behind the concepts themselves.

Given the large amount of literature, there are surprisingly few definitions of TQM. Crosby (1979, p. 58), for example, argues that the word 'quality' should have no qualifiers. He feels that quality 'control' and quality 'assurance' disguise the simple message that quality is 'conformance to requirements' – nothing more, nothing less. Quality management is 'a systematic way of guaranteeing that organized activities happen the way they are planned. It is a management discipline concerned with preventing problems from occurring by creating the attitudes and controls that make prevention possible' (Crosby, 1979, p. 19).

Oakland (1989) stresses the organization-wide involvement:

> TQM is an approach to improving the effectiveness and flexibility of a business as a whole. It is essentially a way of organising and involving

the whole organisation, every department, every activity, every single person at every level. For an organisation to be truly effective, every part of it must work properly together, recognising that every person and every activity affects, and in turn is affected by, others.

(Oakland, 1989, p. 14)

Deming argues that quality is 'a predictable degree of uniformity and dependability, at low cost and suited to the market' (quoted in Oakland, 1989, p. 292), but he rarely discusses TQM *per se*. Macdonald and Piggott (1990, p. 92) argue that 'Quality management is not a fixed body of truths, but a process that is evolving and will take different forms to meet the needs of individual companies'. Many authors emphasize the proactive elements of TQM. Atkinson (1990), for example, says 'TQM is a preventive strategy replacing rework, fire-fighting and crisis management with planning, co-ordination and control . . . [TQM] is the umbrella under which a great number of quality initiatives can be managed.'

One may see a natural progression from quality control through quality assurance and total quality control to Total Quality Management – for example, on the grounds of increasing proactive concern for designing quality in, rather than inspecting it out, and also in terms of increasing comprehensiveness, particularly in regard to the involvement of non-production processes. However, the British Standards Institution sees QC and QA as complementary in its quality spiral (see, for example, BS 5750, Section 0.1, 1987, which suggests they may profitably coexist rather than having a policy of replacing one with the other).

Our analysis of the literature suggests that conceptual models of TQM take little account of other theoretical and conceptual work carried out in areas such as understanding organizations, or the modelling of processes of organizational change. For example, one model of TQM (Crosby, 1979; 1988) argues for wide-scale culture change from a belief in the inherent nature of error, to a philosophy of zero defects. There is considerable exhortation that this should happen; training is used to provide simple problem-solving tools, and there is a detailed, if generic implementation sequence. However, little advice is offered about how one actually secures culture change in different organizations.

The features of TQM can be summed up in the following definition, which we adopt in the rest of the book: *TQM is an integrated, corporately-led programme of organizational change designed to engender and sustain a culture of continuous improvement based on customer-oriented definitions of quality.*

Models of TQM

Most models of TQM have been built from the ground up through the trial-and-error experience of many quality managers and consultants since the 1950s. A high proportion of this work has been based on manufacturing companies – relatively little has been developed for the service sector since the mid-1980s (but see, for example, recent publications such as Edvardsson *et al.*, 1994). Similarly, there has been little critical research. The literature is dominated by three or four particularly influential authors commonly referred to as TQM 'gurus'. How one achieves such status is not clear, but the word signals that much of the writing is promoted with missionary zeal – indeed, those who were trained by Deming, or who were otherwise close to him, were known as 'Deming's Disciples'. There are also half a dozen lesser gurus, some who are relatively recent pretenders to guru status and a whole host of management consultancy-led approaches which have borrowed to a greater or lesser extent from the major writers.

While there is considerable agreement about the general philosophy, there are strong differences in some areas which have led to bitter exchanges between gurus. Macdonald and Piggott (1990, p. 97) cite an article in the August 1986 edition of *Fortune* magazine in which Juran is quoted as saying 'I do not regard Crosby as an expert in the field of quality . . . he is an expert in public relations. He is a combination of P.T. Barnum and Pied Piper.' Macdonald and Piggott go on to point out that Crosby has actually had a good deal more actual practical experience of managing quality programmes than either Juran or Deming. However, Crosby does place less emphasis on statistical methods – something that both the other authors emphasize strongly. Table 2.3 sets out the main steps in each author's methodology.

They all emphasize the need for top management commitment in what are all basically top-led programmes (see below). They also all stress worker involvement and setting up systematic efforts to detect and correct errors. Here Deming and Juran differ from Crosby. They are both statisticians with a concern for the issue of statistical variation. Deming, in particular, insists that one must first understand the nature of variation in a process before making changes. All the authors reinforce the need for continuous effort and the length of time needed to build up a culture of continuous improvement.

Main features of TQM

In the paragraphs that follow we discuss the key elements of most TQM approaches. Differences of content and emphasis between some of the authors of the models are highlighted where they occur.

Staff commitment

Top management commitment to a culture based on continuous quality improvement (CQI) is seen to be essential. This must be demonstrated both by personal commitment and by production of policies and plans which are seen to be consistent with TQM philosophy. CQI must be

Table 2.3   A comparison of the approaches of three key authors on quality improvement

Juran	Crosby	Deming
Build awareness of need and opportunity for improvement	Generate management commitment to the Crosby approach	Create constancy of purpose for continual improvement
Set goals for improvement	Set up quality improvement teams	Adopt the new philosophy
Organize to reach goals – put quality councils, teams and facilitators in place	Quality measurement – identifying current and potential non-conformance	Eliminate the need for mass inspection
Develop and implement training for all	Monitor the costs of quality (i.e. non-conformances)	End practice of lowest-tender contracts
Employ project-based problem solving techniques – use statistical process control but beware of tool-driven approaches	Develop quality awareness in all personnel	Work continually for improvement in every process, using statistical methods
Report progress systematically	Implement a systematic model of corrective action	Institute modern methods of training on the job for all staff
Give recognition where it is due	Plan for implementation of a zero-defects programme	Institute modern methods of leadership based on quality not numbers
Develop and implement systems to communicate results	Define and undertake supervisor training	Drive out fear by encouraging two-way communication
Keep score. Note that quality is not free – there is an optimum trade-off	Zero-defects day: zero defects becomes the performance standard	Break down barriers between departments
Institute a philosophy of annual improvement in all systems and processes	Setting improvement goals within each work group	Eliminate exhortations made without providing methods and systems to do so
	Remove causes of error. Set up a formal system to communicate problems to management	Eliminate arbitrary numerical targets
	Establish explicit recognition programmes	Foster pride in workmanship
	Quality councils – bringing quality people together	Institute vigorous programmes of education and encourage self-development
	Do it over again with a new quality group	Create top management structure to push the above 13 points *every day*

observable in the systems and processes of senior and middle management (for example, in the work of the board or of planning departments), not just in their exhortations to front-line staff. As Peters has argued, the single biggest determinant of a successful TQM implementation is the 'obsessive' commitment of the chief executive and other senior managers (see, for example, Peters, 1989, pp. 70 ff.). The use of the word 'obsessive' reflects the zeal that is held to be required for successful implementations in some American TQM initiatives. Its use would seem to go beyond single-mindedness – it can be almost pathological in its intensity and we believe it is not compatible with the value base of managers and clinicians in the UK NHS. 'Active' or 'total' commitment should be sufficient to describe the requirement.

Corporate planning

There seems to be good agreement that one of the biggest differences between TQM and other quality initiatives is the production of a medium- to long-term organization-wide corporate plan. This must specify the quality dimensions of future strategy by way of a mission statement, goals, objectives and action plans which have an explicit quality orientation. The stress is on top-down corporate planning, though this is increasingly fed by bottom-up information and organizational change as the implementation develops. The planning is synoptic rather than incremental, in the sense that there is a comprehensive planning process for all departments and all levels which are integrated upwards into a corporate plan.

Models of quality appear to be a mixture of forward and backward mapping. These terms refer to the major direction of implementing change. Forward mapping indicates that change is driven primarily downwards and forwards from top management to the consumer. Backward mapping, on the other hand, starts at the point of service delivery, and change is mapped backwards and upwards into the organization from that point (see Chapter 3). Initially, the stress appears to be on forward mapping of quality initiatives as the top of the organization cascades, in a rather prescriptive way, the instructions for setting up the quality system. The form and function of quality improvement groups, for example, are set by the top, though the membership of those groups may be decided at the base. Once structures and systems are in place the top may increasingly encourage the base to backward map by starting with definitions of the external customers' requirements and tracking these back through internal processes to establish customer–supplier chains. Theoretically, there is also an upward-mapping process in which the roles of senior managers and support service specialists are defined by customer requirements. More 'mature' TQM programmes are now increasingly encouraged to engage in upward appraisal of managers by their staff, using customer requirements as the criteria, and major systems redesign using business process re-engineering or business process improvement.

We make the point here that we see a difference in the commercial sector between customer focus and customer empowerment. While all organizations are encouraged to focus on customers, identify their requirements and reorient processes to meet those needs, this almost always remains at the level of focus rather than empowerment. That is to say, customers can only specify their requirements given the information made available to them about the relevant products and services. Since commercial organizations tend not to give customers information which is detrimental to a product, customers often cannot make an informed choice. Any true empowerment of customers would appear to come from the role of what we have called 'informed user groups', including consumer and pressure groups.

Structures for TQM

Almost all models of TQM recommend the appointment of a TQM specialist. This person is variously named a coordinator, facilitator or manager. These terms are applied loosely and the exact role relationships are far from clear. Generally, the post is seen as middle management or senior management in level, with direct access to the chief executive or equivalent. The extent to which there are further posts and groups established varies from model to model. At one extreme, the responsibility for promoting and achieving quality improvements is left entirely in the hands of the existing hierarchies, be they managerial or based on other role relationships. Similarly, issues of quality and proposals for action will be generated within, and be the responsibility of, existing teams, committees and other groupings.

At the other end of the spectrum, a full TQM shadow structure parallels existing ones. In this case, one might expect to find a quality steering group made up of senior and middle managers who may well also meet in other management group settings. Below the quality steering group there will be quality improvement teams, typically made up of middle managers, supervisors and their staff. There will often also be departmental-level TQM facilitators (who are also middle managers) facilitating quality circles or other front-line groups outside their own departments. In all these cases, staff may be members of management-led teams in other working contexts. Where elaborate shadow meetings' structures are set up, it is generally expected that these are only temporary and that they will somehow wither away when operational line managers are fully committed to, and skilled in, TQM philosophy and methods.

Installing separate structures in ways which do not undermine existing line-management chains is more difficult than it sounds. There are many references in the literature to the difficulties for middle managers in TQM programmes (see, for example, Rosander, 1989; Bertram, 1993). They often perceive themselves to be under threat because of the empowerment of their staff, or because those staff may well be working in quality groups which are facilitated by other line managers. This is borne out by our own research in the NHS. It is not unusual to hear of quality groups, particularly quality circles, where the managers of such staff can only attend by invitation.

It should be noted that quality circles are not generally recommended unless they are put in place as part of a much wider TQM process and only after middle management commitment to TQM has been secured. This is based on observations that they cannot make anything other than marginal changes without committed middle and senior managers, particularly when inter-departmental cooperation is required. The Japanese pour scorn on British attempts to introduce quality circles which they see as typical short-term responses to the need to involve workers in problem-solving (Juran, 1988; Rosander, 1989; Macdonald and Piggott, 1990). They would not dream of implementing quality circles until a full supporting structure and culture were in place.

We also note Deming's (1986) observation that some 94% of all faults are designed into the system, and will thus be continuously repeated, while a worker can only influence some 6%. This is supported by Rosander (1989), who has analysed the kind of process improvement which comes from quality circles and shows that, in the main, they are trivial in comparison to the major systems and process issues facing organizations. While this may be true of manufacturing, and also of the pre-delivery processes in a service organization, we would expect that staff involved in actual encounters with users would have considerably more discretion in how the end service is fashioned. However, where problems occur because of a lack of mandate for cooperation between different disciplines or departments, then the extent to which individual groups of staff from any one department can effect changes in the whole process is still likely to be limited.

Process improvement

A major part of the TQM philosophy is a commitment to continuous improvement. All staff, including those in support roles or who are otherwise not in direct contact with external customers, must identify their internal suppliers and customers in 'internal customer chains'. In several TQM models there is then an elaborate exercise in which suppliers and customers explicitly state their requirements so that all parties to a particular process are clear about what is required and what is to be delivered. In other models, this process is more muted, but the end result is still the same. Inter- and intra-departmental groups systematically examine the processes under their control and identify areas for improvement. This is usually accompanied by the setting of standards or targets, which should be a dynamic process. 'Problems' are identified, analysed and prioritized. Action plans are drawn up, implemented and monitored.

Working on the basis of simple supplier–customer chains may be helpful in many manufacturing companies where there are straightforward linear production relationships. However, relationships in service industries are more complex, and nowhere more so than in the NHS. Thus an operating theatre will be both a supplier to, and a customer of, the X-ray department in the same transaction. This is far from just an issue of semantics. The technical and specialist nature of the work means that the X-ray department (the supplier) may well have to dictate its requirement to the theatre (the customer) rather than the other way round.

In our model of quality assurance (Joss *et al.*, 1994), *technical* quality, in this example, may be specified by X-ray, *systemic* quality by the theatre, and *generic* quality by the patient. However, there may be disagreements between all three participants about what would constitute a reasonable waiting time, and between X-ray and the theatre about systemic relationships with each other and with other suppliers. It may well be that the language of supplier–customer chains, with the in-built inference of linearity, is not helpful in these situations. A more useful distinction might be that between service-giver and service-seeker (see for example, Kogan *et al.*, 1971; Jaques, 1976)).

A more useful language may also be that of *transformational* quality (Harvey and Green, 1993). In this case the supplier does not just make a product (as in manufacturing a radio for a customer), or merely add value to inanimate objects (as in repairing the radio for a customer) but, by changing the customer's state, actually transforms the customer. In the case of an X-ray of, for instance, an artery, the product is not just an image; it is also knowledge. This knowledge might be applied to the patient to convince him/her to change diet or exercise behaviour. This is similar to the field of education where an educational institution (or rather its staff) modifies the knowledge, understanding and value bases of the students. The idea of transformational quality can provide important insights into determining quality criteria between competing interests (see Harvey and Green, 1993).

The extent to which agendas for action should be driven by managers or by front-line team members is far from clear. Quality improvement activity must fit in with the general strategic thrust provided by corporate and departmental plans; yet front-line staff 'are the ones who know what the problems are' and therefore must be 'empowered' to contribute to the agenda-setting process in some way. Ways of handling this dichotomy are not well provided for in any of the models we have looked at. Often this is because of a lack of clarity about the roles of middle managers in translating corporate plans into output at the base. It can also be exacerbated by a lack of clarity about the relationship between central or departmental quality staff and operational line managers (see Chapter 8 for our suggestions about how to improve vertical and lateral quality structures in a health context).

Costs of quality (also cost of non-conformance)

The emphasis on this aspect varies, though it is considered to be important. While Crosby (1979) argues quality is free in the sense that it is always cheaper to do something right first time, Deming and Juran are more cautious, with Juran arguing that there is an optimum trade-off between the failure, appraisal and prevention aspects of quality. How authors on quality handle the issue of errors also varies. A distinction is often drawn between errors and defects. The argument goes that people make mistakes all the time. However, if they inspect the work intelligently, make good the mistakes, and (most importantly) trace and eliminate the causes, then the opportunity for defects to occur is reduced. In this sense, a defect is an uncorrected error. However, correcting errors is costly – hence the continuous exhortation to 'get it right first time'.

Crosby argues that the performance standard must be zero defects. He is adamant that 'There is absolutely no reason for having errors or defects in any product or service' (Crosby, 1979, p. 58). Deming and Juran are critical of this standard particularly as the general exhortation is often aimed at junior staff who have little control over most of the factors that lead to defects in work. Deming points to the natural variation in all processes. The key for him is the use of intelligently selected and designed statistical techniques to identify and reduce variation (Deming, 1986).

Macdonald and Piggott argue that the standard is to 'delight the customer by continuously meeting and improving upon agreed requirements' (Macdonald and Piggott, 1990, p. 59). This suggests that if the customer specifies an acceptable level of error, then this is the standard, though one should always be seeking to improve upon it. They argue that seeing the elimination of defects as the driving force behind quality is no longer sufficient to maintain competitive advantage. Even where the technical quality of a product is defect-free, ways can still be found continually to improve presentation, distribution, after-sales service and so on.

Quality of information

For obvious reasons, a premium is placed on the need for high-quality information. Information should be timely and accurate, and meet the requirements of the customer. The latter qualification is an important point – if information is timely and accurate but does not meet the needs of the customers then by definition it is of poor quality. This brings up a fundamental issue which we have observed on several occasions in the NHS: who decides what is relevant about information to the customer? Although the customer would usually be the arbiter of relevance, there are occasions in the NHS where the supplier dictates the nature of information and how it should be used by the customer.

This point has been discussed earlier in connection with process improvement. It can also be a factor in normal working relationships. An obvious example is information about the use of certain drugs, or the relevance of certain tests, where specialist professional and technical staff have a duty to advise doctors and nurses (their customers) on the correct use of prescriptions and tests. This said, the quality of information generally seems to be the key to all staff being able to measure and improve their own performance. It is at the heart of the problem-solving process in quality improvement groups. In the NHS the strength of the purchaser– provider contracting relationship is almost entirely dependent on the quality of information available to both parties. Purchasers have only been able to set measurable standards and targets where information systems are available to monitor them.

Empowering and valuing all staff

While all organisations emphasize how important the staff are, few managers seem to actually put this into practice (for NHS examples, see Dalley and Carr-Hill, 1991). However, the assumption in TQM is that where staff are empowered by being allowed to have a hand in CQI and then rewarded for their efforts, they will be remotivated. Further, since TQM emphasizes the importance of every link in internal customer chains, all staff, including those traditionally seen as of lower importance or status, will have the importance of their contributions brought to notice and explicitly valued. Recognition is a key step in Crosby's 14 steps – see Table 2.3 earlier in this chapter.

Focusing on the customer

It is axiomatic in all TQM programmes that there must be a renewed emphasis on the customer. Considerable effort is expended by commercial organizations in gaining the views of past, current and potential future customers. Reorienting the views of staff about the value of customer complaints is an early feature in many initiatives. While some organizations are content to test customer opinion once or twice a year, there is increasing emphasis on continuous feedback. Post Office Counters, for example, tracks some 20 quality criteria on a monthly basis (see Chapter 6).

Training and education

All TQM programmes stress the importance of education in securing commitment and behaviour change towards CQI. Many programmes that fail during implementation are thought to have done so because of a lack of resources invested in training. (Of course, TQM may also fail because organizations have assumed that training on its own would be sufficient, when fundamental action is usually required in reshaping structures and systems as well as training.) The distinction usually drawn between education and training is that education is about changing attitudes, while training refers to specific tools and techniques for process improvement. Staff at all levels are supposed to be equipped with detailed skills in systematic data collection, analysis and evaluation, though this is biased towards quantitative statistical methods.

The amount of training prescribed in the TQM literature varies, but it is well above what most non-TQM organizations would normally provide, particularly for front-line staff. Oakland (1989) recommends at least 8–20 hours for top/senior management, 20–70 hours for middle management, 30–40 hours for first-line supervisors and 'detailed training' for the rest. This is relatively modest by the standards of many top corporations. The Chief Executive and the other four top leaders of the Wallace Company (a Houston-based industrial distributor) each underwent 200 hours of intensive training on the methods and philosophy of CQI. In another example, the objective of Corning Inc. was, by 1991, to have all employees, over 30,000 of them in 58 locations around the world, spending 5% of their work time in education and training (both examples from TQM Magazine, 1991, pp. 17 and 28).

Even this falls far short of Japanese practice. It is claimed that Japanese employees spend, on average, 22 days of company time per year in education and training, *with an additional 22 days of their own time in further training* (Macdonald and Piggott, 1990, p. 15; emphasis added). The figures do not show the time spent on general job-related technical skills training compared to that spent on CQI methods, though one would expect that the distinction would gradually disappear, as all training is reoriented towards continuous improvement.

Monitoring and evaluation

'Management by fact' is an important feature of all TQM programmes. Thus considerable effort is put into measuring inputs, processes and outputs of key organizational systems. In TQM this goes well beyond production processes. Thus one might find personnel clerks monitoring the quality of handling of personnel files using internal customer-based criteria such as accuracy of entries, currency, turn-round time, and relevance to users. Quality assurance systems would be in place for parts of the organization as different as vehicle maintenance and the staff canteen.

A different issue altogether is the requirement to evaluate the progress of the TQM implementation itself. This 'meta-evaluation' is an important feature of successful TQM programmes and was conspicuously absent from most of the TQM pilots in our NHS research sample.

Achieving a TQM culture

The overall requirement of a TQM programme is to develop a 'TQM culture'. This should actively encourage the breaking down of inter-departmental and inter-disciplinary barriers in order to improve communication and encourage joint approaches to problem-solving. For example, Ford and IBM both say that they wasted years before realizing that most quality improvement opportunities lie outside the natural work group (Peters, 1989, p. 76). One of the myths about Japan is that TQM was successful only because of workers' subservience and loyalty to their organizations. Nothing could be further from the truth. The early days were marked by fierce hostility between competing groups of workers who blamed each other for problems of poor quality. One of the reasons for developing the notion of internal customers was to try to break down strong divisions between different departments (Ishikawa, 1985).

One of the consequences of systematically turning the spotlight on processes where there are weaknesses may be to exacerbate inter-departmental differences which have lain dormant, or which have been accommodated by negotiation. This phenomenon has been serious enough for Neuhauser (1988) to liken it to 'tribal warfare'. If TQM is really going to take hold as a culture, it is argued that the organization must overcome these barriers and become one of open learning, where all staff are able to accept, offer, and act upon constructive criticism from others.

Authors on TQM suggest that quality must become everyone's business, not just the business of management, or those working in specialist QC, QA, or TQM roles. TQM should be implemented organization-wide – in personnel, finance, administration, marketing, planning, research and development, estates management, and catering – not just in production.

The idea behind CQI is that the search for process improvement should be relentless and continuous by all staff. The Japanese have become the proponents of encouraging hundreds and thousands of small incremental improvements rather than large set-piece organizational changes. For example, in 1960, Toyota's suggestion scheme raised less than one suggestion per worker per year, of which only a third were implemented. By 1982, it averaged over 30 suggestions per worker per year (1,905,682 in total), over 95% of which were acted upon (Peters, 1989).

Target and standard setting should be a dynamic process where there is continuous review, not a static process of setting standards that staff already know they can achieve. When standards are achieved they should be immediately challenged in terms of searching for further improvement. This brings about more uniform definitions of quality across all the functions and departments in an organization, as staff increasingly focus on their customers' requirements (though operationalizing common definitions may take different forms in different departments).

Translating manufacturing models of TQM for the service sector

Generally speaking, the private sector service industries were slow off the mark in getting into TQM when compared to manufacturing. Indeed, when they did begin to engage with the issue of quality, much work focused around modifying concepts of QC and QA from the manufacturing sector and applying them to services. This was often supported by customer relations awareness training for staff, in recognition of the importance of customer contact. However, research in service quality since the early to mid-1980s has demonstrated a number of differences between the nature of manufacturing and that of the service industries (see, for example, Edvardsson and Gustavsson, 1991). The differences have been sufficient to suggest that the transferability of manufacturing models of TQM to the private sector services may be limited.

In manufacturing, TQM was primarily seen as a vehicle for reducing the variation in production processes – a 'do things right' product orientation. This is in contrast to the customer- or market-oriented service industries which have a concern to 'do the right things'. Whereas reduction of variation may also be of concern in service-delivery systems (for example, in getting the buses to run on time), a simple process improvement approach may work less well in personal services such as banking, hairdressing or health services. Here, it seems to us, the stress should be on increasing variation by emphasizing the individual needs of consumers and therefore increasing the skill repertoires of staff so that they may more appropriately meet wide variations in demand. As Rosander (1989) has persuasively argued, one of the problems of TQM is that every customer is a sample of one. The consequences of this are that simple analysis of aggregated quantitative data derived from processes may be insufficient to explain customers' requirements. He argues that there should be continuous monitoring of the qualitative aspects of current customers, potential customers and lost customers.

There are other differences which flow from this analysis. For example, the production of tangible goods allows for quantitative measures of quality, since these can be monitored throughout the production cycle and in later use. However, in service delivery, much depends on the qualitative aspects of staff–customer encounters. In these, the service is 'consumed as it is constructed', and there is often little to show for it after the event. It may be that assuring quality in these circumstances requires different methods of monitoring and evaluation. Whereas QA systems in manufacturing may emphasize conformance to the technical requirements of internal customer chains, with only oblique references to the end user, the staff–customer encounter depends entirely on participation by the customer. Monitoring quality in this process, therefore, appears to require feedback from consumers (individually and in aggregate) on a *continuous* basis.

One should also note that as products and services become increasingly sophisticated and complex, the proportion of service content in work appears to go up. This is so both internally to the organization, as in research and development, planning, system design, personnel and finance, and externally in customer support. Thus, even where an organization is primarily preoccupied with the production of particular goods, it may find itself having to provide a range of services to support sales of the goods – for example, the opportunity to test the goods before purchase, training of users in the use of the product and after-sales service, perhaps throughout the life of the product. A typical example is in the area of computer hardware and software.

Furthermore, the percentage of people who work directly in service provision as opposed to manufacturing organizations is steadily increasing. US census figures show that it is now around 75% and, as Deming points out, this is an underestimate, since it does not include those staff in manufacturing organizations who are actually employed in service-provision aspects of the business (Deming, 1966, p. 184).

Recognition of some of the differences between product and service arenas has led, since the early to mid-1980s, to a rapid increase in the search for alternative models of service quality – models that would help understand the issues at the conceptual, design, implementation and evaluation stages. Much of this work is at an early stage of development but appears to offer promising alternatives to the application of manufacturing models of quality. Chase and Bowen (1991) have suggested that these research efforts are based on three basic theories. The first is attribute theory, which assumes that service quality is primarily dependent on the attributes of the service-delivery system. In this case, managements have considerable control over the processes of ensuring quality, and models drawn from the world of manufacturing (Crosby, Juran and Deming) may be applied for that purpose.

Customer satisfaction theory is very different in that it assumes that service quality is defined with reference to the customer's perceptions of what constitutes quality, with this, in turn, being dependent on the match or mismatch between the customer's expectations and his or her actual experience of the service (see, for example, Parasuraman *et al.*, 1985). The third approach, interaction theory (see, for example, Klaus, 1985), emphasizes the importance of the customer–employee service encounter itself.

As work continues in this rapidly expanding field, more elaborate models are being developed which overlap the three categories above. From the early work by Gronroos (1984) on the relationship between functional quality (how the customer gets the service) and outcome quality (what the customer gets), researchers are now looking at comprehensive blueprinting of processes (Shostack, 1987), expanded marketing models (Bitner, 1991) and culture-related models which take issues such as value structures and the referent groups of a target customer population into account (Edvardsson and Gustavsson, 1991). It is likely that further developments in this field will lead to very different models of TQM from those currently relying on models originally developed for manufacturing industries. As we shall see in the next section, the NHS, in particular, requires rather different approaches to TQM.

The health sector

Changing definitions of quality

TQM might be seen as a set of ideas whose time had come, given the changes in management and direction of the NHS since the early 1980s.

However, there is still a major struggle going on between the dominant pre-1980s culture and more recent attempts to shift towards a managerialist and consumer-oriented culture. As we have previously noted, Pfeffer and Coote have called for a 'democratic' model of quality which would better meet the broader welfare goals of equity and responsiveness. Their approach would recognize the differences between commercial and welfare transactions, and the multiple roles played by different stakeholders. This model would also require very different kinds of managers from those currently working in many parts of the UK public sector. Under the democratic model managers would need the skills to manage decentralized units with devolved powers, including budgetary management. They would need a blend of technical, professional and management expertise, and an openness to consumer empowerment rather than consumer focus.

This links with the notion of post-bureaucratic management (Hoggett, 1991) and has led to discussion about a 'new public management'. Smaller self-contained units with flat organizational structures, containing a high proportion of professional staff, working in self-managed teams, may well be increasingly common in the new world of purchaser–provider contracting. The relationships between these groups and consumer-driven quality form an important part of more recent literature (see, for example, Gaster, 1991).

The requirement for a whole new range of management skills and a change in the value systems of both managers and professional staff have been of central concern to training and personnel professionals in the NHS since the Griffiths reforms were first mooted (Thompson, 1992). Distinguishing the pre- and post-Griffiths cultures, Harrison *et al.* (1989) summarize the older culture as one where:

(a) the organization was not unitary and where management was not the major influence;
(b) the organization was largely reactive in nature, with little in the way of formal forward planning (though we note attempts to install complex planning machinery from 1974 onwards);
(c) the pattern of change was incremental and at the margins, with the value of the status quo largely unquestioned; and
(d) the organization was producer-oriented rather than consumer-oriented.

The early 1980s saw a stream of government initiatives aimed at securing a paradigm shift within the public sector services generally – greater concern with value for money, devolution of responsibility to local levels, and attempts to shift from administration of inputs to accountability for managing process and outputs. Concurrent with these moves were calls for more responsiveness to consumers' views and the provision of greater choice. Considerable support for these views was provided by the Griffiths (1983) report. The report pointed to some of the weaknesses of consensus management; to the lack of accountability, particularly for proactive planning and securing change; and to the fact that there was little real and continuous evaluation of performance with regard to both efficiency and effectiveness; it suggested that the NHS was too far from its consumers.

Less strongly voiced were considerable concerns behind the scenes about the escalating costs of an increasingly 'high-tech' service, and a growing elderly population which consumes a disproportionate amount of resources. In addition to the increased demands from a more elderly population, we can also expect difficulties in resourcing that demand because of deepening problems of staff recruitment and retention, caused by the demographic trough (see, for example, Tuckman and Blackburn, 1991). These resource concerns are significant because, by and large, they are avoided in discussions within the NHS when issues of quality are raised, although they are common enough in discussions about NHS funding in general. Indeed, there have been strong moves to decouple quality from efficiency. Where they are connected, it is in the context of value for money.

In contrast, advocates of TQM argue that there is gross waste in both manufacturing and service organizations – claims of anything from 20% to 40% of operating costs being held to be directly or indirectly attributed to unnecessary waste (Crosby, 1979; Atkinson, 1990). There is less evidence available for the public service sector (but see Koch, 1993, on studies in the NHS which show that similar savings are possible; and also Joss, 1995).

One should be clear that TQM is concerned with unnecessary costs incurred through errors, not cost improvement programmes that make cuts across the board on the grounds of economy alone. While managers might have to make the political decision to distance themselves from the cost improvement programmes in order to gain the cooperation of clinicians (Pollitt, 1990, p. 444), they cannot ignore waste and errors if they are serious about implementing TQM.

Early NHS documentation on QA programmes made little or no mention of the savings that could be generated through the introduction of QA programmes. For example, Duncan Nichol's first major circular to regional general managers in June 1989 (EL[89]/MB/114) speaks about the importance ministers attach to the 'quality of care and the provision of a service which is sensitive to the needs of its customers' (para. 1). To this end they wanted each DHA 'to ensure that its units develop systematic, comprehensive and continuous quality review programmes' (para. 2). The focus would be on medical audit, the Waiting List Initiative, and quality review mechanisms in every unit (para. 3), with four specific initial areas for quality improvement – appointment systems, information to patients, hospital waiting and reception areas, and customer satisfaction surveys.

Even in more recent statements, quality was coupled with value for money and identifying consumers' needs, rather than with scope for explicit reductions in wastage (Merrifield, 1990a; 1990b, Waldegrave, 1991). This resonates with the broader definitions of error within TQM since, for example, if one provides a service that is poorly used because it does not meet clients' needs, this would be construed as an error, notwithstanding that the input resources and processes are in themselves of 'high' quality. This value-for-money-type approach is more acceptable than searching for more blatant examples of waste caused by sub-standard work or wasteful use of materials.

Decoupling issues of quality from the need to make more efficient use of resources has allowed NHS units to reverse the normal priorities inherent in manufacturing models of TQM. For example, in the course of defining three components of quality as 'customer quality', 'professional quality' and 'process quality', Øvretveit (1990, p. 132) has observed that:

> It is the process quality element of health services which has been largely ignored in discussions of quality assurance and quality programmes, but which is central to most commercial organizations' strategies ... doing the right thing, right first time, and every time, and the systems to support staff in doing this have proved extremely successful in commercial companies.

This point was not lost on some of our NHS interviewees who had previously worked in industry. As they observed, the rationale for implementing TQM in manufacturing normally has the following priorities:

(a) Get it right first time, every time; tighten up on the systems; eliminate waste; reduce the need for post-production inspection; reduce the overall cost of the product. This will also improve product quality.
(b) Generate a climate within production processes of an obsession with continuous improvement and the elimination of error. Widen this to all parts of the organization – personnel, finance, administration, marketing, etc. Build the so called 'quality culture'.
(c) Become more responsive to customer demand and reorient all processes and procedures towards satisfying the customer.

These priorities had been reversed at many TQM pilot locations. Although 'get it right first time, every time' did appear in some mission statements and aims and objectives, the emphasis was quite muted, except at some sites which were explicitly following Crosby-like approaches. Of importance here is that the applicability of manufacturing models to the public health sector may be significantly reduced when the priorities are reversed, since the main rationale in manufacturing is for a major focus on elimination of waste in production design and management.

Manufacturing models provide relatively little advice about how to design mechanisms for improving the staff–customer encounter, for empowering the user, or for improving access or equity. It could be argued that it is unfair to expect the models to do this since they were not designed for it. It would be equivalent to expecting a service-encounter model (see, for example, Klaus, 1985), which focuses on improving the service encounter at the point of delivery, to improve the quality at earlier stages in the process. Even without the considerations above, one might expect private sector models of QA and TQM to meet considerable difficulties in transferring to the NHS. The models have been generated within, and rely on the context of, manufacturing industries which have markedly different characteristics to public sector health services. These are summarized in Table 2.4.

The cultural differences are most marked when one looks at attempts to define quality in a health service context. Much of the early work was by the American doctor, Donabedian, who has been publishing since the mid-1960s. He has been particularly influential in the UK with his structure–process–outcome (SPO) model which has been adopted by many health authorities (Dalley and Carr-Hill, 1991). More recent and accessible references are included in the References (Donabedian, 1980; 1982; 1988). His basic proposition is that the assessment of quality must take into account the attributes of the setting of health care provision including human and financial resources, facilities, organization of those resources, and methods for evaluation and monitoring (structure); what is actually done in giving and receiving care, including both practitioners' and the patients' contributions (process); and changes in the health status of patients as well as improvements in their understanding and their satisfaction (outcome).

Steffen (1988) defines quality in terms of its capacity to achieve stated goals. He also emphasizes that any definition of quality must include an assessment of the patient's goals and values. Both Donabedian and Steffen distinguish between the medical aspects of the physician's contribution and those aspects which revolve around the physician's inter-personal skills (or lack of) in handling socio-psychological issues which may well also involve a patient's non-medical goals.

However, the extent to which these definitions of quality are in keeping with models of TQM is doubtful. First, there is a strong focus on the physician–patient relationship. The contributions of many other actors receive little coverage. TQM would emphasize the importance of all other contributions – not just as static, one-off inputs, but rather their sequenced introduction at different stages of a process. TQM would suggest that the doctor almost always depends entirely on these contributions for effective performance.

Second, both authors suggest that high-quality care can be held to have been provided irrespective of the outcome. Donabedian (1988) writes:

> Even if the actual consequences of care in any given instance prove to be disastrous, quality must be judged as good if care, at the time it was given, conformed to the practice that could have been expected to achieve the best results.

Steffen (1988) makes a similar point:

> I locate quality in the capacity to achieve a goal (the outcome) rather than in the outcome itself. Thus the capacity to achieve a goal may have been inherent in the medical care given but for various reasons

Table 2.4 Some differences between private sector manufacturing and public sector health

Features	Manufacturing industries	Public sector health
Structure and culture	Strongly top-down, management-driven, often with a tradition of corporate planning and proactive management. Profit-oriented and used to being in a highly competitive internal and external environment.	Decision-making process through issue-specific, multi-disciplinary groups of administrators and autonomous professionals negotiating consensus, (although this should not disguise the strong hierarchical nature of relationships, e.g. nursing). Process of change often diffuse rather than top-down or bottom-up. Welfare-oriented and mainly non-competitive, though they increasingly compete for resources. Reactive rather than proactive.
Systems	Experience of quality control (QC) with probably some elements of quality assurance (QA) in place, at least in production. Performance indicators (PIs) geared towards output, though mainly still financial. Higher productivity or increases in sales rewarded by increase in profits which may or may not be shared with staff. Strongly costs-oriented even in specialist departments like personnel, marketing and sales. Not necessarily good IS/IT, but at least some experience of managing on the basis of (mainly quantitative) information.	Little experience of QC and QA except in few areas such as X-ray, pathology and medical engineering. PIs based on administration of inputs and quantity of outputs. Other than promotion, no history of personal financial incentives or performance-related pay (PRP). Perverse incentives operate whereby improvements in productivity (e.g. treating a greater number of patients at lower cost per patient) are penalized by lack of commensurate increases in overall funding. No systems for managerial or financial accountability in medical specialisms. Poor information systems and technology (IS/IT).
Staff	People have been recruited, trained, motivated and rewarded on basis of output-oriented, profit-driven culture. Have management and financial skills and experience to draw on.	Most people in organization still from era when welfare and service aspects dominated. Not primarily motivated by profit or efficiency motives. Apart from specially recruited managers, most higher level staff used to

Table 2.4 (Cont.)

Features	Manufacturing industries	Public sector health
		administrative or professional lines of control – little or no performance management training or experience.
Customer base	Customers could use purchasing power to switch to alternative suppliers who are realistically available in most areas of business. Quite well informed about desirable aspects of goods and services but not so likely to have knowledge about less desirable aspects.	Customers use the service because they have to, not because they want to (illness not being a sought-after condition), although this may be less relevant in the case of proactive health care. Little or no freedom of choice for most people. Poorly informed about services as consumers.

this capacity was blocked and the goal was not achieved. Still quality care was given.

Williamson (1991, p. 20), on the other hand, argues that this view cannot be sustained any longer.

> If we are to progress we must have better outcome measures than those presently available. It is clear we must have some condition-specific clinical outcomes against which to measure success, not merely the absence of mortality or morbidity. In addition though, we must try to develop an understanding of the patients' psychological and social functioning, their general level of well-being and their perceived health status. We no longer accept the defence 'the operation was successful but the patient died'; in future we have to reject the plea 'we did everything possible but the patient is still complaining about this and that'.

A further influential model of quality in health care has been proposed by Maxwell (1984). This, too, seeks to broaden the criteria by which one might judge quality, away from narrow manufacturing or process-oriented models. He argues that there are six dimensions – access to a service, relevance to need (for the whole community), effectiveness (for individual patients), equity (fairness), social acceptability, and efficiency and economy. These dimensions have been helpful in taking stock of services at a macro level, but they have proved less helpful in defining the more pragmatic aspects at operational levels (see, for example, Brooks in her introduction to Sketris (1988); and also Evans and Corrigan, 1990, who had difficulties in using Maxwell's dimensions when trying to develop a standard for multi-disciplinary discharge procedures).

Carswell and McAlister (1991) have suggested that we may need to recognize a 'mezzo-context' which relates to the service provided to aggregates of people at the institutional level. This might bridge the gap between the macro and micro approaches discussed above. This echoes our suggestion that quality criteria must be specified for at least six different levels of organization (Chapter 4).

While recognizing the differences between these approaches and those of private industry, attempts have been made to integrate them. The Royal College of Nursing, for example, which is now 'committed to promoting the concept of TQM' (RCN, 1991, p. 1), quotes the British Standards Institution definition of quality (RCN, 1991, p. 10), describes the contributions that Crosby (1979) and Oakland (1989) can make (RCN, 1991, p. 2), and suggests that these approaches should be carried out within a Donabedian-like framework. For a model of TQM in practice, the booklet draws on Mobil Corporation's Exploration and Product Division TQM programme. Somewhat surprisingly, Maxwell's dimensions, particularly those of accessibility, equity and relevance to community need, are not discussed, though his work is cited as further reading. It is of some concern that the fundamental differences in these different approaches appear to have been ignored by the RCN.

Realistically, operationalizing mixed models in this way will face problems. A major difficulty will be attempts to widen medical models of quality assessment to include managerial criteria. Clinicians already feel under threat with the move towards a market philosophy which is underpinned by an increase in managerialism and a diminution in the power of professional groups, particularly medical staff. TQM promises to give managers, who are perceived as being equipped (at best) with a set of diffuse general skills, a set of 'theoretical' and conceptual models which they can use to develop expertise and so challenge the professionals (Tuckman and Blackburn, 1991).

Pollitt (1990) sees the main implications of introducing QA as being twofold – explicit public statements about standards of service provision (thereby demystifying and delimiting the technical criteria used for medical judgements of quality), and an increased responsiveness to the stated or implied needs of users. He puts forward six possible relationships between managers and professionals in relation to QA. These range from minimal intervention at one end of the spectrum, through to a point where the professional is directed to employ a designated approach which is then driven by the management in such a way that results would affect the pay and other rewards of the professionals concerned. The six approaches are set out in Figure 2.3.

Pollitt (1990, p. 442) advises a middle course (approach 3), perhaps with some requirement that the data be made available for, and be of a kind that would allow, inter-institutional comparison. While this might be

Figure 2.3 Pollitt's (1990) variations on manager–professional relations in a QA implementation

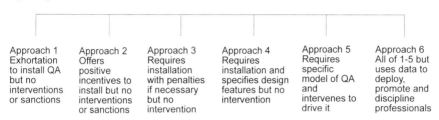

Approach 1 Exhortation to install QA but no interventions or sanctions	Approach 2 Offers positive incentives to install but no interventions or sanctions	Approach 3 Requires installation with penalties if necessary but no intervention	Approach 4 Requires installation and specifies design features but no intervention	Approach 5 Requires specific model of QA and intervenes to drive it	Approach 6 All of 1-5 but uses data to deploy, promote and discipline professionals

appropriate for the specification of a single QA system, it would probably be seen as insufficient within a full TQM programme across a unit. For example, one could envisage each of six or seven clinical directorates deciding to design and implement their own versions of QA with little in the way of coordination or compatibility. For an ideal-typical or orthodox TQM programme, there might well be pressure for Pollitt's fifth approach. This would be one in which there would be more management intervention in order to ensure that a generalizable corporate approach was being taken. Here managers might be involved in the full specification of the design, development, implementation and monitoring of any systems for continuous quality improvement. The role played by the general manager or chief executive would then be one of coordinating and integrating multidisciplinary relationships between all those involved in process improvement at senior levels.

In our argument for a mixed model of quality assurance for the NHS (see Chapter 8) we have argued for a position in which the centre would require all services and departments to put QA systems in place, but work with the services to develop systems which would be most appropriate to those services' requirements. The role of the centre would then be in carrying out a 'meta-evaluation' of how well those systems were operating, and each service would also be required to evaluate the content of its own work. This requirement, on balance, would most closely approximate to Pollitt's approach 4, with approach 5 being a last resort.

Other quality initiatives

When any organization decides to introduce TQM, it will be faced with the issue of how to integrate ongoing initiatives (quality or otherwise) with the main TQM thrust. The NHS is no exception. A study in 1989, when the first of the TQM experiments were just starting, identified 1,478 separate specific quality initiatives under way at that time in England and Wales (Dalley and Carr-Hill, 1991). The extent to which so many initiatives can be integrated into a comprehensive and coordinated TQM approach at a pilot site will depend on several factors. Some initiatives might be directly related to quality improvement, for example quality circles, whereas others might contribute to improvements in quality more indirectly, as in resource management or contracting. Clearly, those that have direct QI goals will be easier to reorient towards TQM goals than initiatives which only have QI as a subsidiary goal.

Initiatives might also be classified as one of three kinds, according to their scope. The first would be *national* initiatives, examples of which might be TQM, the Resource Management Initiative, medical/clinical audit, purchaser–provider contracting, and RCN-based standard-setting initiatives. (National standards which affect non-clinical services, for example hygiene in catering, and which are applicable throughout the NHS would also fall into this category.) The second category would be *district/unit*-wide projects such as seeking hospital or BS 5750 accreditation, or a multi-disciplinary group looking at building quality into a new hospital. The third category would be *departmental* exercises such as looking at waiting times in a clinic, or improving the standard of meals in a canteen.

Obviously it will be more difficult to integrate a national exercise with TQM than a ward-level project. The most difficult exercise of all could be predicted to be a national requirement which is only loosely connected with the principles of quality improvement implied by a particular model of TQM. This has been most apparent in a number of the initiatives sponsored by the Department of Health which have caused difficulties for TQM sites. We carried out an analysis of some of these initiatives for the Department in 1992, and a comparative table from that piece of work is included as Appendix I. Of course TQM was only an experiment at a small number of NHS sites and NHS-wide initiatives could not be expected to be modified to take account of this. However, if TQM is going to be adopted on a broader basis, the issue of integrating existing and new initiatives so that they are consistent with any particular model of TQM is going to be crucial to its success.

As discussed earlier, change in the NHS up to 1980 was largely incremental (Harrison *et al.*, 1989). Our experience has also been that it has been relatively uncoordinated and without a long-term sense of continuity in strategic thrust. This has led to many staff believing that changes are 'flavour of the month' in character, with current initiatives heading progressively for the back burner as new ones come along. One might expect, therefore, that an initiative like TQM which is supposed to be 'for ever' and which is held to be the over-arching rationale for all other organizational activity, would tend to be bolted on to earlier initiatives rather than acting as the unifying force. Here we outline some of the key features of the national initiatives from a perspective of the extent to which they sit easily alongside the broad principles of TQM.

Resource Management Initiative

An important development introduced from 1986 onwards was the Resource Management Initiative (RMI). This was designed to 'enable the

NHS to give a better service to its patients by helping clinicians and other managers to make more informed judgements about how the resources they control can be used to maximum effect' (*NHS Management Board Bulletin*, August 1988). The RMI process has many of the features of a TQM initiative. It requires commitment of personnel; devolution of authority; multi-disciplinary collaboration; managerial support; and an implementation strategy (Buxton *et al.*, 1991). Where RMI is weakest in TQM terms is the extent to which internal and external customers are built into the process of development and review.

Audit approaches

Medical audit is another important plank of the government's drive for QA. It is defined as the 'systematic, critical analysis of the quality of medical care, including the procedures used for diagnosis and treatment, the use of resources, and the resulting outcome and quality of life for the patient' (Department of Health, 1989). Again, the test of medical audit is if it can be comprehensive enough to take account of the contributions of all participants to a total patient episode (including the patient). During the period of our study, medical audit was viewed as being a doctor-driven process in which other staff and patients played little part, but there have been encouraging moves more recently with the introduction of clinical audit. This is beginning to integrate various forms of audit, including nursing and therapy practice, and provides an opportunity to take more account of patients' views and the total patient episode (see Kogan *et al.*, 1995a; 1995b).

Williamson (1991) distinguishes three forms of audit: *professional audit*, which includes evaluation of services provided for a disorder and depends on the exercise of medical judgement and the judgement of other professionals; *clinical audit*, where there is an evaluation of other elements of services provided in relation to a disorder, but which does not rely on the exercise of professional judgement; and finally, *service audit*, which relates to aspects of the case unrelated to the disorder. While this is helpful in establishing procedures and accountability, it denies the inter-relation between the three areas. For medical audit to meet the principles of TQM it would have to be geared more towards process audit. This has been recognized by the Department of Health, which is promoting a move away from medical audit towards a broader-based clinical audit system. The need for integrated service audits is covered in more detail in Chapter 8.

Standard setting

Standard setting, which is a natural precursor to any audit process, has made a valuable contribution to quality improvement activity but falls some way short of TQM for the following reasons: first, it is uni-disciplinary; second, it is often confined to single departments, particularly nursing;

third, it is not integrated with corporate planning; fourth, it is unconnected with the general strategic thrust; fifth, it tends to be a static process rather than part of a dynamic system (even where implementation has followed the RCN's Dynamic Standard Setting System approach); and finally, it is often focused on a narrow set of standards rather than on the whole field of possible process improvement.

BS 5750

A number of trusts have opted for BS 5750 registration for some of their services. This is a registration process in which set QA systems are inspected and validated by inspectors from the British Standards Institution. It is quite possible that a TQM programme in an organization may pursue BS 5750 registration for some of its processes and systems. However, that would not be a sufficient condition for TQM. TQM is the total management system within which BS 5750 might form one element. BS 5750 validates the QA arrangements for a given system or set of systems using criteria set by the organization. It says little about the viability of an organization (it could go to the wall the day after certification). Nor would it say much about the appropriateness of a particular process in terms of meeting, for example, Maxwell's criteria of access and equity (unless the organization decided that it should, in which case it would have to have QA systems in place to demonstrate that these criteria could be assured).

BS 5750, on its own, is seen by many to be incompatible with TQM because of its lack of focus on the end user. Where suppliers are part of a supplier – customer chain of producers and manufacturers, the internal customer's specifications will often form the basis for the QA standards. However, there are many 5750 systems in place which do not take account of the end user's requirements. It is not unusual, for example, for NHS bio-medical engineering departments to have secured BS 5750 registration but have standards in place which are unrelated to patients' or carers' needs. It is theoretically possible that one could secure BS 5750 for an extremely good QA system that assured quality based on unprofessional, unethical or otherwise low standards.

Summary

The following are the main points in this chapter:

- Commercial quality systems originated in manufacturing. They began with a principal concern to improve quality by focusing on *technical* aspects of production. More recently they have begun to encompass *systemic* and *generic* issues.
- Manufacturing models of TQM have been adapted for the private service sector. They may be appropriate for improving 'pre-service' delivery processes but may be inadequate for improving the service encounter

itself. Service quality models have not found their way into the literature on TQM in health in Britain until very recently (see Øvretveit, 1992).

- Many contrary definitions of quality abound in the literature and definitions in the health arena are particularly hotly contested. There are few analytical or comprehensive definitions of TQM. It tends to be defined by a catalogue of characteristics which are held to be essential for its implementation. We define it as *an integrated, corporately-led programme of organizational change designed to engender and sustain a culture of continuous improvement based on customer-oriented definitions of quality.*

- Many studies talk about the need to empower consumers, but at the outset of our research there was little evidence to suggest that this aspect had found its way into the operational consciousness of managers or clinicians at acute units, though some aspects of community services were further ahead in this respect. Providers had chosen to rely on post-episode satisfaction surveys, many of which were designed, carried out and analysed solely from the providers' perspective.

- The strong emphasis on patients and other users did not seem entirely consistent with the top-down, forward-mapping style of planning and implementation which was evident in the NHS when we began our evaluation. Often, it seemed, the senior managers decided for themselves what the users and the staff wanted. It was only when the implementation was in its stride that the organizations started seeking staff and patients' perceptions of their needs.

- By and large, models of TQM are generic in the sense that their proponents apply them to a wide range of different organizations, yet they draw little on the broader organizational literature and are particularly thin on how to operationalize TQM in different organizational cultures. A combination of exhortation, education and a few simple diagnostic tools is expected to bring about widespread organizational change.

- A wide range of other quality improvement initiatives is being implemented at the same time as TQM, but few, if any, meet the principles of TQM. Little work has been carried out on the integration of managerial and professional perspectives on quality improvement, including models of audit.

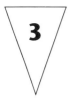

3 Designing for quality

Introduction

Most writing about quality is stronger on what to do than on how to set the right conditions for doing it. Those who wish to implement Total Quality Management successfully usually find they must change organizational working and styles. TQM is, indeed, intended to achieve wide-scale organizational change.

The initiatives which we have observed display a wide range of assumptions about ways in which change might be formulated and implemented. The complexity is compounded by the fact that these attempts are taking place alongside changes of momentous importance to the NHS. The role of the district has changed from that of management and ownership to that of purchaser and strategic planner. A shift of services from residential provision and, to some extent, from acute units to the community also involves substantial changes in structure and relationships. Alongside the formally established changes are the growing power of such concepts as 'the customer' and 'empowerment', and these are reinforced by the introduction of contractual relationships. The implementation of organizational change is, indeed, a continuation of political processes in another arena (Rein, 1983).

Models of change

The Department of Health TQM initiatives were intended to cause change in culture, organization and working practice. They were also intended to test ways in which change might be implemented. Many of the classic theories of change and implementation came to life in the actual events observed in quality programmes being tried out in the NHS and in our two commercial research sites. It may be helpful to specify some of the concepts which illuminate the kind of organizational issue relevant to the installation of quality systems. Here is a list of some of the more useful formulations:

- top-down and bottom-up modes of change;
- backward mapping and forward mapping;
- normative and operational modes of working;
- normative re-educative and coercive strategies;
- rational organization and political bargaining;
- managerial and collaborative modes;
- socio-technological factors;
- markets and contractual arrangements.

We will now consider these in terms of their relevance to the NHS quest for quality.

Top-down and bottom-up modes

A phrase often used of TQM is that it is 'top-led and bottom-fed'. This evokes previous thinking about the extent to which an initiative should be 'top-down' or 'bottom-up'. Such thinking emerged in the context of earlier changes in the NHS by Hunter (1983) in his consideration of the centre–periphery and periphery–centre models applied on that occasion to the relationship between the central government departments and health authorities. He noted the paradox of health administration in which a balance has to be maintained between certainty which demands control, and flexibility which is a prerequisite of innovation. These considerations affect our notions of change and endure today.

The top-down model assumes that only the top, the directors of a trust and the management team, are in a position to take sound allocative decisions. A bottom-up model relies on the belief that service innovation requires groups to collaborate within trusts or managed units. In the latter model, the top has a facilitating as much as a control function. Top-down approaches are assumed to inhibit rather than promote innovation at the periphery because policy-making and implementation are interactive processes. A bottom-up model may assume pluralism and aim for consensus through learning, rather than compliance and control.

In our fieldwork we noted these as real issues. In a small number of cases, management had led strongly, and most operated on a top-down model, but had not secured the belief and commitment of those at the operational levels. In these cases the initiative either remained at the level of training and raising of consciousness, or produced formal compliance which faded as soon as the prime mover had moved elsewhere. Where mission statements had been developed by top management in virtually a command form, these had emerged either in different forms or not at all at operational levels.

In other examples, bottom-up initiatives were started by individual departments and wards without explicit support from management. Such initiatives might lack legitimation and resources, place intermediate levels of management in ambivalent positions, and be weak in terms of inter-departmental connection. Issues could then arise about the capacity of the whole unit to demonstrate that it had a firm grip on quality issues, as is indeed required through the new contracting systems and through the more general traditions of accountability to the public for the services which they would purchase.

In TQM, therefore, the sequence of introduction and implementation becomes a prime concern. 'Top-led and bottom-fed' attempts imply an iterative process in which the 'top' formulates its policies on quality only after it has created a joint agenda with those working at the base. It does not begin to move towards the more formal description of requirements, standards and conformance until it has recruited the support of the operational levels. Only once that is done is the 'top' able to move more firmly along the lines of a TQM implementation in which all of its components, including the organizational and setting of standards, can be included.

Backward and forward mapping

A further format of the top-down, bottom-up conceptualization refers to implementation in terms of 'backward mapping' and 'forward mapping' (Elmore, 1982). Forward mapping is the traditional implementation process. It assumes that objectives are set by policy-makers at the top of the organization and that implementation is achieved through the phased application of specific techniques. Backward mapping, however, starts from the point of service delivery. The point of analysis is where practitioners meet their clients. It then works sequentially through the various organizational actors until the traditional top of the policy process is reached and policy then formulated and confirmed. In most of our sites there was little evidence of any form of mapping, either forward or backward, but the general organizational pattern was one of forward mapping.

As suggested above, the top-down and bottom-up formulations can be linked to the idea of backward mapping to produce a rolling or helical process to promote the notion of 'top-led, bottom-fed' change (see Figure 3.1).

First, the top of the organization decides it intends to pursue some form of TQM. The bottom could make such a decision, but not have it mandated, and there need to be connections made with other operational units. In this sense one must always start such a programme in top-down fashion. However, this approach embodies a period of consultation with staff, patients and other users to establish their expectations and requirements.

This is followed by a backward-mapping exercise to analyse the capacity

Figure 3.1   Helical arrangements for balancing top-down and bottom-up modes

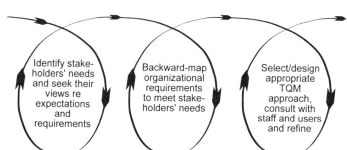

of existing systems and processes to meet these requirements. It is only then that the top decides the most appropriate way to move forward. Even then it continues to consult the middle and the bottom about proposed changes. As we shall see later, this is a long way from what we observed in either the concepts or implementation of TQM in the majority of the sites evaluated for the TQM experiment. How such an approach might be achieved is discussed in more detail in Chapter 8.

Normative and operational modes of working

Some further theoretical underpinning for the negotiative pattern implied by the model suggested above can be found by consideration of the dual modes of working by different entities within organizations. The work of actors in a multi-level organization is framed by two dimensions of working. One is that of levels – central authorities, unit, department, individual, for example. The other concerns modes of working – the normative and the operational (Burns, 1977; Becher and Kogan, 1992).

In the normative mode an individual responds to certain values and norms which might derive from training and education, a personal belief system, and connection with professional groups outside the employing organization. These values also respond to some extent to environmental pressures. The operational mode concerns the tasks which must be performed. In practice the normative and the operational are inextricably bound up – the performance of a task or a function is undertaken with values forming at least 'a field of force' (Lewin, 1952).

The norms are likely to be different at each level of a professionally based organization and will need to be negotiated. Thus the concerns of individual practitioners working with patients ought not to be in conflict with those of managers of systems, but they will occupy different 'assumptive worlds'. The performance of tasks at the different levels is held together by allocations, managerial authority and other forms of rule setting. The holding together of the normative modes at the different levels is undertaken through evaluation and other forms of normative influence.

Acknowledgement of the legitimate differences in norms would be the basis for a combined top-down, bottom-up mode of change and action. Most models of TQM demand conformity to collective definitions of quality. This may conflict with the value systems that guide different professional staff. The extent to which NHS units do in fact develop approaches that can span the breadth of professional and non-professional opinion is taken up in Chapter 5.

Rational and political bargaining processes

Yet a further dichotomy in implementation is that between rational organization and processes of political bargaining. While for purposes of analysis these might be thought about separately, in practice they are usually inseparable. That is to say, even the most 'hard-nosed' rationalistic process of implementation is likely to succeed better if it involves discussion and negotiation with the main stakeholders in a change process. This was most obvious at one of our TQM pilot sites, where the ideas of one particular writer on TQM were being pushed through with little or no discussion. The consequences were predictable – lack of support, poor motivation, loss of confidence in the Chief Executive and little or no movement below senior management levels.

Wolman (1984) considers implementation to be primarily a rational process which can be divided between the formulation and carrying-out phase (that, again, is often an artificial distinction in practice). It is often assumed that where failures occur they occur in implementation. But in Wolman's view the quality of the formulation and conceptualization, such as the creation of control or training or other structures, is as important as, or more important than, the quality of the implementation itself. This analysis is consistent with the increasing effort in industrial TQM settings to apply TQM to the design and development stages of production processes (see Kackar, 1985). Certainly it is not unusual to find commercial organizations spending anything up to a year in the planning stage of a TQM initiative. We would identify lack of thought at these stages as responsible for many of the weaknesses in the NHS TQM initiatives.

This stage would require considerable expenditure of time and effort in analysing customers' needs and the capacity of the organizational culture, structures, systems, processes and people to meet those needs. If the programme design is not adequate for analysing the problems to be tackled, or for accommodating political problems, or for tackling technical feasibility and the unintended consequences of change, then failure is likely to ensue.

Managerial and collaborative modes

A further variation of the top-down and bottom-up models can be found in contrasts drawn between managerial and collaborative modes (Burns,

1983) and change caused by external as opposed to internal agents. Coercively administered forms of change, embodying the use of sanctions, are contrasted with collaborative modes which depend upon incentives.

Normative re-educative and coercive strategies

There is also theoretical work on ways in which individuals or groups can be persuaded to change. According to Chin and Benn (1969):

> Normative re-educative approaches to effecting change bring direct interventions by change agents, interventions based on a consciously worked out theory of change and of changing, into the life of a client system, be that system a person, small group, an organization or a community.

Such approaches assume that the culture will move forward towards open learning and dynamic self-correction. They emphasize the involvement of clients in programme change and bringing clients and their problems into 'dialogic' relationship with the way in which the problems are seen by the change agent.

On the face of it, such educative change models start at the periphery or with the individual and take account of psychological and other needs. They are, nevertheless, compatible with managerial leadership which might be seeking normative re-educational methods to further organizational goals. Thus while individuals are given the opportunity to internalize and work out organizational goals, this would be a different process from that implied in Hunter's centre–periphery model in which the knowledge and power of individual practitioners at the periphery are the primary motive force in securing change throughout a larger system.

In the case of the TQM experiments it was not easy to reconcile professional or technical with systemic and generic notions of quality because the different versions of TQM were not fully conceptualized before they were launched and existing forms of quality assurance had not been adequately analysed. These seem to be minimal conditions for launching ambitious normative-re-educative initiatives. Nor could coercive strategies have succeeded, if only because regions, districts and trusts had not usually implemented TQM at their own levels and existing relationships and leadership had been weakened by the purchaser–provider split.

All of the theories cited so far address two interlocking sets of questions. The first concerns the organizational or institutional structures through which action is legitimized and control is exercised. Here the issues are of authority, accountability, power and use of sanctions and organizational rewards. But, secondly, the theories carry with them assumptions about what constitute the best ways of inducing organizational change and learning among individuals and larger groups. Some models might start from this second set of issues, but they inevitably travel through the same terrain. There is a continuing connection between questions of authority and questions of how to engage commitment and gain consent to change.

Policy and planning process

Other classic formulations of the policy process and its implementation reflect the influential analysis set up by Braybrooke and Lindblom (1963), in which they distinguish between synoptic planning and piecemeal planning or 'muddling through'. Synoptic planning assumes that an organization can make a wholesale analysis of the needs and requirements it must or should meet and can convert these broad objectives into working programmes which can then proceed on rational lines. The intellectual process is deductive, that is to say starting with large propositions about the human condition and deducing from those the actions and principles that must be brought into operation.

The opposite process, of muddling through, is not only incremental but also disjointedly so. From this perspective, 'disjointed incrementalism' is the truly rational and practical way for actors to proceed. In such a process, the conceptualization is inductive, for inasmuch as overriding policies are necessary they are induced from a range of experiences in the field. The actor faces the here-and-now reality and reacts to it in a rational fashion. To some extent it is possible to reconcile the two approaches inasmuch as the here-and-now reality can be framed within at least a middle-term plan which might be changed as experience demands.

Again, this is a key issue for TQM. The expectation is that senior management must provide constancy of purpose (Deming, 1986) through developing and then sustaining a long-term vision of the changes necessary to install a 'quality culture' – a process that is held to take anything from five to ten years to secure. The top must also drive the implementation through a series of set stages (see, for example, Crosby, 1979) which demand long-term, organization-wide planning and action. If, however, as Braybrooke and Lindblom suggest, implementing change is actually a piecemeal exercise, responding mainly reactively to changes in the environment, then TQM must find some way of bridging corporate action with the reality of day-to-day management at the base.

In our study we found that tensions were generated by the requirement of a corporate approach in trusts and directly managed units where the value of diversity was entrenched in multiple occupational cultures. Yet there seems to be good agreement that TQM entails the production of a medium- to long-term organization-wide corporate plan which will specify the quality dimensions of future strategy by way of a mission statement, goals, objectives and actions plans which have an explicit quality orientation. We found a corporate drive for quality in only a small number of the NHS sites where we worked (see Chapter 5).

Socio-technological factors

Some important insights can be derived from functionalist theory as applied to working organizations (see, for example, Woodward, 1965). This concerns ways in which organizations are and should be fashioned according to the fit between the culture and the purpose of the organization. The organization is thus a function of its 'socio-technology'. This means that the organization is fashioned to meet the nature of the task. From that are derived the working relationships which underpin the more formal structures.

The relevance of this to TQM in the NHS is strong. The dominant culture has been that of the health service practitioner prescribing for, and treating, the individual patient as a unique set of problems to be solved. Professionalism is primarily individualistic, whereas planning and organization are intrinsically collectivist. In the professional model, standards are inculcated through training and consensus reached within the many individual professions within the NHS.

TQM, however, seeks to promote collective dimensions of quality – that is, to characterize elements of quality in terms of requirements and standards and, indeed, to quantify them so that degrees of non-conformance can be established. The rendering of account would thus be easier. It also seeks to move from the traditional altruistic but unilateral relationship between professional and client, towards the empowerment and participation of the client as an equal partner in the securing of his or her own health.

A similar theme is pursued by Schön (1983). He contrasts a model of practice based on technical expertise with one grounded in reflective practice. The former assumes a fully competent expert who keeps his or her distance from clients and requires deference and respect for the professional *persona*. In contrast, the reflective practitioner demonstrates that he or she is still learning, does not require the maintenance of an occupational façade, and is prepared to negotiate joint meanings in interactions with empowered clients.

There will always be tensions in any major change programme since, almost by definition, it will require shifts in the purpose of the organization. This will bring those who propose the change into conflict with the old order. One of the key issues for proponents of TQM, therefore, is to identify how and where these conflicts will occur and fashion the changes in such a way that they accommodate, as best they can, the expectations and requirements of key participants to the process. For example, in the NHS many groups already possess professionally fashioned concepts of quality. It would be a poor TQM system that does not fully respect and accommodate them.

These assumptions are partly social or political but also partly technical. In terms of inputs and processes, one must ask what modes of change best support and encourage changes in the organization's socio-technology. Specifying approaches which match or develop the appropriate kinds of staff attitudes and skills is an important consideration. So, too, is the need to develop information systems for TQM which are achievable given the current state of technology. The traditional approach to individualized patient care has meant that, in the past, information has normally been kept on a case-by-case basis and not easily aggregated in the form required for TQM-type process improvement. We have seen difficulties that sites encounter when the demands of TQM are not matched by the skills of key staff or are let down by the technology needed for implementation.

It is also necessary to be able to specify the key outputs and outcomes. However, these depend on understanding the relationships between processes and outcomes. Processes by which people become ill or get better are not as clearly understood as many would hope. Since TQM depends on a better understanding of processes (managerial, administrative and medical), these processes must be capable of better specification.

Not surprisingly, it is a lot easier to define administrative processes than medical processes. However, if TQM in the NHS is to get beyond improving administrative processes (though our observations are that this in itself would be a considerable advance) those involved must begin to tackle the complex issues of specifying desirable medical outcomes and linking these, causally, to antecedent processes. What will lead to the best health states? Once that is determined, different social relationships ensue and the structures are conditioned accordingly.

Theories of evaluation

Many of the developments under the TQM banner draw attention to recent changes in assumptions about the evaluation of service. In the course of what has been described as the 'rise of the evaluative state' (Neave, 1988; Henkel, 1992), it has been noted how under previous versions of the welfare state, evaluation was essentially *ex post*. That is to say, the service providers were trusted to formulate the statement of needs and negotiate for funds, and any evaluation of outcomes would take place afterwards, and often in a somewhat unrigorous fashion.

By contrast, in these sterner times, evaluation is conducted *ex ante*. That is to say, there is rigorous scrutiny of the objectives of services within cash limits which are determined mainly according to what can be afforded, rather than the needs of the service being funded. The evaluative frame is thus established from the very beginning and inputs are carefully scrutinized, as are the potential outputs and outcomes. Again, TQM responds to this move inasmuch as it seeks mission statements and objectives as the first line upon which TQM can be administered.

TQM also demands detailed analysis of systems and processes in order that a case for change can be justified in advance. It is, perhaps, unique, in that whereas recent moves to evaluate have placed the evaluative power outside the systems being evaluated (as with the strengthening of national inspectorates in the social services and the operation of the Audit

Commission), TQM in a sense brings (as it is intended to bring) the processes of the evaluation back deeply into the working process and into the hands of those most directly concerned with doing or managing the work.

Markets

The metaphor of the market is widely used in the NHS, largely to describe the newly formulated purchaser–provider division. What in fact results is not a market in the full sense. In a free market each individual is expected to optimize his or her own advantage. The aggregate of individual decisions to buy and sell will create services and goods through the mechanism of supply and demand, and will ensure that new goods are developed by providers. It is obvious that the new contracting arrangements fall short of the full market concept in several ways.

First, they do not provide a personal profit motive, although institutional and job survival may be considered an adequate substitute. This will be an important consideration for the debate about performance-related pay.

Second, the purchasing decisions are not made by the ultimate customers, who have no direct purchasing power, but by their professional proxies.

Third, the feedback from provision to market demand, and with it the demand for new goods and services, must rely on second-order mechanisms such as patient satisfaction surveys which are as yet not a good alternative to market research. The more important element of the changes consists less in their market characteristics than in the creation of explicit contractual arrangements which provide for analysis of quantity, quality and cost and for forms of *ex ante* evaluation.

The essence of the new arrangements is less that they rely on market behaviour than that they set up tighter demands and expectations through the use of contracts for quantity, quality and timeliness. Contracts are conceptually separate from markets.

In reflecting on these theoretical dimensions, all of which are familiar to students of organization, we noted that some decisive choices seemed to be entailed in the adoption of the major TQM models. Our own estimate, as we began our study, was that the complexity of the NHS was such that all sides of these theories would run together and reach compromises.

We shall be returning to some of these organizational constructs when we consider requisite models for TQM in Chapter 8.

Summary and conclusions

How might an effective model of TQM take these theories into account? It should

- seek to identify the relevant strengths and developmental needs of the system, processes and resources, including people and the requirements of all its stakeholders;

- move into a bottom-up model of implementation as soon as possible through staff attitude surveys, newsletters, open forums and the like;
- develop a model of TQM which recognizes both organizational needs and socio-technology; that is, a matching of the structures to the tasks being performed;
- in designing TQM, capitalize on the skills of professional staff;
- set up systems for continuous monitoring of customers' requirements, expectations and satisfaction;
- train all staff through programmes that respect individual skills and interests;
- subscribe to a model in which the centre provides advice and direction on broad strategic lines but allows units and departments maximum freedom to develop quality improvement systems appropriate to their needs.

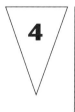

4 Evaluating quality to improve services

Setting out the issues

There are many approaches to quality improvement, but we will be focusing here on the evaluation of QA and TQM because they are the most elaborate versions of formal systems for quality improvement. TQM, in particular, encompasses most, if not all, of the features of other approaches and therefore requires one to consider the widest range of issues when thinking about how to evaluate quality.

Evaluation and measurement

Although the terms 'evaluation' and 'measurement' are often used interchangeably, they are actually quite different. Measurement refers to the process of obtaining a score for some variable. Evaluation, on the other hand, is making a judgement about performance. The distinction is important because making a judgement entails recognizing the influence of personal and organizational value systems in evaluation. Suchman (1967) pointed out that the evaluation process is a circular one which begins and ends with value judgements. An adaptation of his model is shown in Figure 4.1.

It would, for example, be a relatively simple matter to measure how long ophthalmology patients wait for operations. We would have to agree the precise definitions of when waiting began and ended but the actual measure (time) would be easy to agree, to count, and to analyse. However, evaluating the overall effects of a programme designed to reduce waiting times would be much more complex. The programme might reduce waiting time to operations but increase the waiting time to appointment. On

Figure 4.1   The circular evaluation process

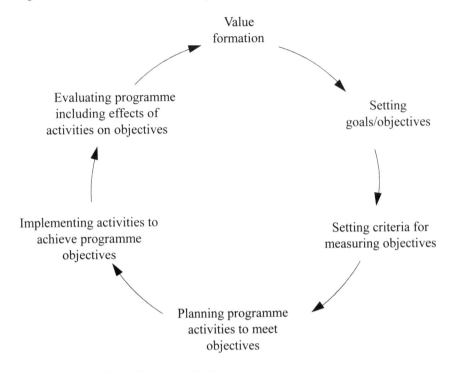

Source: adapted from Suchman (1967)

a technical level, this could adversely affect prognoses or increase the rate of misdiagnosis. It might also increase costs or divert resources from other important work. What should the balance be between economy, efficiency and effectiveness? What about the effects on patients' perceptions, and how much weight should we attach to them? This would be a matter of judgement and would almost certainly produce different views among the key stakeholders.

Evaluation and measurement of TQM

Evaluation of quality in the private sector has traditionally been seen as relatively uncontroversial since definitions of quality have been simplified and well agreed. The issue has been seen as one of how to improve quality not evaluate it. However, as the discussion above has suggested, evaluating quality in a public sector service is rather more complex.

The same can be said of measurement. The choice of what to measure, how to measure it, and how to make sense of often conflicting data from different sources, involves giving a good deal more attention to the whole issue. This is particularly important in all quality improvement approaches because a cornerstone is the emphasis on systematic measurement.

We should also note at this point that the Health Service has by and large relied on qualitative measures. This has been particularly so when looking at medical matters. However, evaluations need not be quantitative, and when one is looking at issues of quality it is probably more helpful to use a mixture of qualitative and quantitative measures.

TQM has tended to focus on process improvement and customer satisfaction. Also, until more recently, most effort has been put into measuring performance at lower levels in organizations, principally at the interface with customers. However, since quality improvement is a feature of all successful organizations, whether or not they are doing TQM, one should really be asking the question 'What is the added value of formal QA or TQM?'

At this point one moves from measuring a particular variable into making a judgement about the value of the results. An important distinction is also made between evaluating the quality of services and evaluating the extent to which a particular model of quality is being followed. The latter is an area on which many organizations have put little emphasis, preferring to evaluate quality improvement on a range of often narrow process or output criteria.

However, an organization might secure technical improvements in the quality of a product or service at the cost of adverse effects on wider issues including staff morale, environmental pollution or longer-term customer dissatisfaction. We have also noted in our research that while a particular model of TQM is being pursued in order to facilitate process improvement, other organizational changes – for example, restructuring or new reward systems – are implemented in ways which are not consistent with the TQM approach being followed. How one defines the criteria by which quality improvement will be judged is therefore a crucial issue. This is taken up in more detail in the next section.

In this chapter we look at designing evaluations at both the working and at the total organizational level. We have not set out to provide an exhaustive guide to methods of evaluation or measurement – there are already a number of useful and easily obtained general publications (see Appendix II). But we look at some of the issues which need to be considered when evaluating QA and TQM in a public sector service organization such as the NHS.

We have divided the discussion into five areas – *what* to evaluate, *where* to evaluate, *who* should evaluate, *who* should be evaluated, and *when* to evaluate. The last two issues depend on an analysis of the first three. These can be viewed as a three-dimensional matrix (see Figure 4.2).

It can be seen that it is possible to conceptualize a single quality measure, or an entire evaluative system on these three dimensions. For example, one might ask a patient how satisfied he or she was with the way an appointment was made in order to evaluate that person's perceptions against

Figure 4.2   The relationship between who, what and where in the evaluation of quality

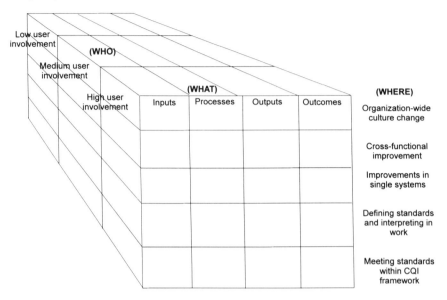

a set of written standards for appointments. This activity would fit in the cell of Figure 4.2 as identified by the coordinates high user involvement – processes – meeting standards.

However, if the purpose was to review a skills mix system which was designed to match nursing qualifications and experience with the complexity of cases, one might be concerned with the cell labelled medium user involvement – inputs – single system. As a final example, one might want to examine the effects of senior management meetings on organizational culture (low user involvement – outcomes – organization-wide change).

For evaluations to be consistent with the principles of TQM we would be looking for them to encourage high user involvement wherever possible and focus primarily on processes and outputs/outcomes. Again, although evaluations might focus on a single organizational level, a full programme of evaluation should be reviewing performance at all levels.

The implications of Figure 4.2 are discussed in more detail below. However, it is important to note at this stage that traditional evaluations have often been limited on all three dimensions. As far as *who* is concerned, there are few examples of high user involvement in designing or applying measures, or in redesigning services following evaluations – something that we believe should be a key feature of TQM in a public sector organization.

In terms of *what* to evaluate, the traditional focus in the NHS has been mainly on *post hoc* accounting for inputs. More recently there has been a shift towards analysing processes and their immediate outputs, but longer-term work has been dogged by difficulties in designing health outcome measures. The issue of *where* to evaluate has followed the tendency in the commercial sector to concentrate efforts and resources on measurement of service delivery at the interface with internal and external customers. However, a comprehensive evaluation of TQM should also look at the impact of TQM on structural, cultural and systems issues at higher levels in the organization.

What to evaluate in QA and TQM

In part, what to evaluate will depend on the features of the particular model of quality being followed. As discussed in Chapter 2, we have defined TQM as an *integrated, corporately-led programme of organizational change designed to engender and sustain a culture of continuous improvement based on customer-oriented definitions of quality*. On this basis a successful TQM initiative could be said to have the following features:

- dynamic and sustained senior management commitment to TQM;
- integrated planning for operations and quality at all levels;
- methods and systems for systematic measurement and evaluation of quality improvements;
- organizational structures for quality improvement to ensure accountability for quality and support for staff in their quality improvement efforts;
- education and training for all staff in quality improvement methods to create a highly skilled and motivated workforce;
- staff empowerment to enable the maximum contribution of all staff to continuous improvement;
- movement towards a common definition of quality based on customer requirements;
- an organizational culture of continuous quality improvement.

These features will normally be translated by an organization into measurable objectives with associated measures and action plans. The objectives would then serve as the basic criteria by which one would evaluate a TQM implementation. However, evaluators cannot always rely on an organization having a comprehensive or consistent set of objectives. Further, there may be important weaknesses in the relationships between the objectives or in the logic of their implementation. For this reason it is often valuable to have an independent evaluation undertaken by outside experts who can bring a broader and more objective perspective to the implementation.

Since we have argued that quality has three important and quite distinct dimensions – *technical*, *generic* and *systemic* – we feel that evaluations should take account of all three areas. It is important to note that these three dimensions are not the same as those based on the perceived requirements of competing stakeholders, although there are obviously important inter-relationships. For example, Øvretveit (e.g. Øvretveit, 1992) has developed a system for improving the quality of health care based on three dimensions of quality – *professional*, *client* and *management* quality. In his terms, *professional* quality is based on 'professionals'' views of whether professionally assessed needs have been met using correct techniques; *client* quality is whether or not direct beneficiaries feel they get what they want from the services; and *management* quality is ensuring that services are delivered in a resource-efficient way.

At first glance our term *technical* might be read as Øvretveit's *professional*, our *generic* as his *client*, and our *systemic* as his *management*. However, there are important differences. The first is that Øvretveit's 'stakeholder' model implies that each group is the referent on quality for that area – thus only doctors can legitimately speak on professional quality, managers on resource allocation and patients on service satisfaction.

Clearly, there are circumstances when only a doctor could comment on the technical aspects of some cases. However, there are many areas of medical practice that could do with a healthy 'injection' of consumer voice. In our model of quality we would want to extend the role of consumers to participation in the evaluation of all aspects of services provided by both providers and purchasers. We return to this issue in our discussion of who should be doing the evaluating later in this chapter.

The third consideration under the heading of what to evaluate is at what point one should be evaluating – at the input, process, output or outcome stages as shown in Figure 4.2. The traditional focus in the public sector has been primarily on inputs – for example, proper accounting for money, staff hours, goods and other resources. Commercial models of QA have shifted the focus towards process improvement determined by user-based definitions of quality, and the NHS is beginning to follow suit. However, because definitions of quality of health outcomes are problematic there has been a tendency in the NHS to focus on evaluating quality of service delivery against professional views of what the user wants in terms of stages of the process or immediate outputs.

Most authors conceive of the stages in input–process–output–outcome fashion, although there are variations. Donabedian's (1980; 1988) influential model, for example, provides for three stages – structure, process and outcome. In his terms, *structure* is a comprehensive set of input issues including human and financial resources, facilities and matters of structure and organization; *process* includes the process of giving and receiving care; and *outcome* refers to both changes in health status and patient satisfaction.

We should clarify how we are using the terms 'outputs' and 'outcomes'. We take outcomes to be of broader significance than outputs, and more the longer-term result of an input–process–output chain. Technically, however, there are outcomes of each stage of any input–process–output chain. For example, the stating of objectives, whether it be clear and cogent or in muddled fashion, is an outcome of TQM effort. The processes by which

Table 4.1 Outcomes from the processes of a TQM implementation

Process outcomes	*Result if outcome is not achieved*
Awareness of TQM programme	TQM will be a non-starter
Understanding of TQM	Staff may well be aware without understanding
Commitment to TQM	Staff may understand without being committed
Acquisition of problem analysis and measurement tools	Staff may be committed without having the skills to change
Appropriate individual changes are applied to problems as a result of proper data collection and analysis	Staff may be committed and skilled but not engage in behaviour change. Change may also be based on unreliable information
Cross-functional process improvement takes place through negotiating agreed requirements within customer–supplier chains.	Change may only take place within small processes and then break down because of poor interfaces with other key departments/functions
Desired change takes place on organization-wide basis	May only take place in some lead departments
Continuous improvement is sustained and becomes a way of life at all levels – the so-called quality culture	TQM will always be a time-limited project, not 'for ever'

different forms of quality assurance are installed and implemented may produce greater 'empowerment' at the operational base and some enfeebling of the authority of middle management. These, too, are organizational outcomes of TQM.

Although each model of QA and TQM has its own preferred methodology, most follow a similar sequence for implementation. In Table 4.1 we list the main stages of a general TQM implementation and the possible outcome of failing to complete each stage. It can be seen that each stage depends to a large extent on a satisfactory outcome from the previous one. It is therefore a sound idea to develop a system of evaluation which will identify the outcomes of each stage. In our evaluation of the Department of Health's pilot TQM projects we selected criteria for evaluating the projects in this way. The main criteria we used to evaluate these projects are shown in Appendix III (see also Joss *et al.*, 1991, for a more detailed discussion about the choice of criteria). These criteria were designed to cover input, process and output/outcome issues at all levels in units concerned. They included outcomes that should have been observable from changes in:

- *inputs* – benchmarks derived from an analysis of the context facing the site; resource requirements for improving quality; the resulting objectives and plans; construction of a coherent model for change
- *processes* – results of corporate planning; multi-disciplinary process improvement; continuous monitoring of processes
- *outputs* – committed and knowledgeable staff, including senior management; moves towards a common definition of quality; improved quality planning; empowered staff and consumers; evidence of reduced multi-disciplinary barriers; identifiable process improvement; and increased customer satisfaction.

It is important to note that the act of setting criteria, in itself, changes the context within which a site will operate. The criteria publicize the required changes and people will take up positions with respect to them. Where they are received positively they can be used for a variety of purposes. Several of our NHS TQM project sites, for example, used these criteria in order to evaluate their starting positions and their later progress. Note that the criteria covered both general features of TQM (i.e. progress on implementing TQM structures and processes) as well as specific gains made in improving the quality of service.

Where to evaluate

As we have already observed, most effort in quality programmes goes, not unnaturally, into measuring quality of service at the base of the organization, particularly in relation to the interface between staff and external customers. This is then supported by improvement activity in operational processes that immediately support service delivery at the base – hence the references to notions of 'internal customers'.

As TQM progresses, process improvement activity is extended laterally to non-operational support services such as finance, personnel, administration and so on, and nowadays, much new emphasis is being placed on issues of structure, culture and the design of systems. The current fashionable emphasis on 'business process re-engineering' is an example of increasing concern about how to realign organizations to changing customer requirements. Much of the effort goes into asking fundamental questions about the nature and purpose of the organization and its systems. Rather than asking the question 'How can we improve this system?' one might be asking the question 'Why do we do it this way at all?'

Our view would be that process improvement activity needs to take place at all levels in an organization. Further, this activity should be directly related to the key results areas of people working at each level. In a number of instances in both the public and private sector we have seen senior managers exhorting those below, especially at the base, to improve the quality of their work seemingly without any appreciation of the fact

Figure 4.3   Operationalizing TQM at different levels in an organization

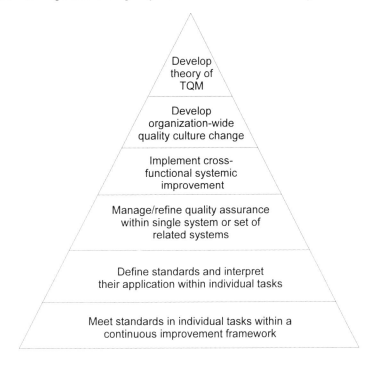

Develop
theory of
TQM

Develop
organization-wide
quality culture change

Implement cross-
functional systemic
improvement

Manage/refine quality assurance
within single system or set of
related systems

Define standards and interpret
their application within individual tasks

Meet standards in individual tasks within a
continuous improvement framework

that senior managers are also equally accountable for improving the quality of work at their own levels.

If the theories and concepts of TQM are to be translated into effective and continuous quality improvement activity at the base then the ideas must be operationalized at each level. Figure 4.3 shows one way of describing the requirements at different levels based on the ideas of Jaques (see, for example Jaques, 1976; 1989).

Some of the features of working at each level and the implications for evaluation are discussed below. We discuss some of the differences and give examples at each level, although there is no doubt that exceptions to our general examples could and should be tried. While specific evaluations could be carried out at any level, a full programme evaluation would almost certainly have to look at relevant issues at all the levels.

The first two levels

Starting at the base of the pyramid, we can say that the work at the first two levels is mainly concerned with delivering appropriate services in individual cases. The work is about fashioning a response to individual need – in this sense each case is taken as unique. Evaluation here will be focused on whether or not standards of care were met in specific cases. In our quality model, this would cover generic and technical issues although the implications of systemic matters might be taken into account in considering the effects in any particular case. Any evaluation should assess the extent to which senior management rhetoric is being converted into behavioural change in the key areas that are specific to each level.

The third level

The third level is concerned with quite different work. Principally it is about matching resources to changing patterns of demand, where the demand is considered as flows of work over time. This requires that cases are aggregated in some way and analysed using common criteria – for example, the average time required to treat a particular group of cases. At this third level it is perfectly proper to apply quantitative measurement techniques to aggregated cases.

The use of basic descriptive statistics can be helpful in gaining insight into the way flows of cases have been handled. For example, in a study by Bell *et al.* (1993) an analysis of chiropody patients' responses to 16 statements about important features of the service showed that 15 out of the 16 were positively viewed by over 78% of respondents. Over 90% thought that they were treated with respect, had clean and tidy surroundings and so on. However, the survey indicated a problem with follow-up appointments – only 47% knew after their appointments when the follow-up visit would be. This shows the value of quantitative analysis when looking for trends or problems which are common to the cases in a particular sample.

More sophisticated statistical techniques, including statistical process control, have been specifically developed for analysing work at this level. However, quantitative measures such as this are not helpful when monitoring or evaluating the quality of service at the first two levels, when one is concerned primarily with individual perceptions. This is graphically illustrated in the Bell *et al.* study where, in the same survey, several patients stated they had difficulty walking because of the length of growth of their toe-nails between four monthly visits.

Clearly it is of little comfort to these patients to know that they were in a minority and that an overwhelming majority of the sample were highly satisfied with their treatment – as Rosander (1989) has remarked, when it comes to quality of service, 'customers are in a sample of one'. There is no substitute for staff talking to *every* patient, not a sample, about their individual problems and looking for alternative ways of meeting their requirements. Where problems appear to be common to a significant proportion of patients with a similar condition, then it might be the time to apply quantitative statistical techniques.

This, incidentally, raises another problem associated with the design of survey instruments. It is common for designers to interview samples of potential respondents using unstructured interview techniques to identify common themes for later development as questionnaire items. While this is perfectly proper, one wonders what happens to those idiosyncratic worries which never make it into popular concerns.

Evaluation at the fourth level

This is the level at which managers and professional staff are accountable for cross-functional process improvement, and one would expect to find performance measures in place for activities which are appropriate to this level. People at this level should be accountable for systemic quality issues such as reducing inter-departmental barriers and facilitating cross-functional process improvement activity. They should also be accountable for generic quality issues. These might include such features as chairing effective meetings, keeping their promises, and being accessible to all staff.

As far as evaluation is concerned, this level may also be amenable to quantitative techniques. However, the work is rarely straightforward enough to treat as relatively unconnected streams of activity which can be analysed into simple trends. For example, the issue of blood samples arriving at a laboratory with incorrect or illegible labels could be analysed at one level as a lack of care, time, handwriting skills, or any number of other factors. The incidence of inadequate labelling could be plotted by frequency, and subjected to statistical process control and other sophisticated techniques. This may well be sufficient to identify apparent causes and suggest appropriate corrective action.

However, the issue may also be underpinned by more abstract concepts that concern broader issues such as communication, professionalism, morale or motivation. Poor communication, for example, will almost certainly be the result of a complex set of inter-related factors which will not normally be amenable to simple interpretation – indeed, one of the reasons for enduring poor communications in organizations is the tendency to apply simplistic corrective action to extraordinarily complex phenomena. At this fourth level one might require the ability and the necessary technological support to model complex phenomena of this sort in the search for comprehensive integrated solutions.

The fifth level

At this level one is concerned with creating an environment whereby a culture of continuous improvement can be engendered and sustained throughout the organization. People working at this level should be drawing on models of organization and relevant social, political and economic theory to develop organization-wide changes which are coherent and internally consistent.

Much emphasis would be on the development of the organization's values and work should be under way to integrate appropriate leadership behaviours with broad-based systems changes. Recent work has also shown the increasing importance of symbols and symbols change in developing new cultures (see, for example, Macdonald *et al.*, 1989; Hammer and Champy, 1993). Any evaluation of TQM would probably start with collection of base-line data on the current quality culture and current state of quality of services across the organization, but interest at this fifth level would be on

- the relationships between the base-line data, senior management's perceptions about quality issues, and the reasoning behind the choice of any particular model of TQM,
- an analysis of structures and systems for planning, installing and evaluating TQM in terms of the models of change implied by the arrangements, and the extent to which they appeared to meet identified needs of staff and customers;
- the coherence and internal consistency of objectives, targets, and plans for future changes in the light of proposed mission and/or value statements about quality.

The sixth level

Here one is concerned with generating policy at regional and central government level. Those working at this level should be developing, and making arrangements to test, more refined or completely new conceptual models of quality improvement for the NHS as a whole. These would go well beyond traditional or orthodox arrangements for TQM and would take into account new theoretical work in related fields of social policy.

Who should be involved in evaluations?

Commercial TQM approaches exhort companies to 'identify their customers' requirements' and 'meet customers' expectations', but there is little evidence that many of them go as far as actually empowering customers by involving them in setting or measuring standards, or in redesigning services when they fall short of the required quality levels. Partly this has to do with maintaining competitive advantage. Few companies are prepared to discuss their shortcomings with their customers and it is difficult to see how they could remain in business if they were to tell current or potential customers that better alternatives were available elsewhere.

The question then is 'Should it be different for public sector services?' We believe that it should, though we can see how this will cause difficulties for provider units working in a quasi-competitive market. For example, how long could a provider stay in business if it were to advise patients to go to another unit where better-quality services were available? While the answer, in the longer term, is to improve services to the level of its competitors, the provider has a conflict of interest since its funding is dependent on numbers. Where will it get the money to invest in improving services if it turns away business?

There is a range of possible ways to involve users in evaluation. As we have already argued, we would not want their contribution to be limited to providing information about their satisfaction with just the generic aspects of quality after they have received a service. It is important that ways are found to involve service users and other stakeholders in health care (parents, relatives, professional carers, local citizens) in the design, delivery and evaluation of services.

The involvement of users will also depend on which mode of quality we are considering – technical, generic or systemic. If we compare Øvretveit's dimensions of quality with ours, we get a 3 × 3 matrix which can be used to analyse the potential involvement of different stakeholders (see Table 4.2). The table shows that all the stakeholders have at least some contribution to make to every area. Of course, there are many difficulties associated with building users into the evaluative process. These include the issues of competence, confidentiality, commitment and reliability.

Informed user groups

The issue of competence can be tackled, in part, through the use of what we have called 'informed user groups'. These are groups of people with a common interest in either a particular unit (say, an acute hospital or community unit) or a condition or range of conditions (as in the case of a coronary support group). There are already many such groups in existence, although their relationship to the respective units has often not been clearly defined or agreed.

While many of these groups now get good information about a medical condition from both purchasers and providers, it is still rare to see them built into service planning or evaluation in any systematic way. The exceptions tend to be the larger national groups such as the National Association of Women and Children's Hospitals which has been influential in securing many user-driven changes in, for example, maternity services. Many user groups have developed when sufferers of a particular condition, or their carers, get together for mutual support. We would see a wider variety of people getting involved in the evaluation process through broader-based groups of this kind.

Other sources of competence that can be drawn on include local researchers and other academics with interests in evaluation or health issues. Community health councils are also an obvious source of skills. Since the late 1980s, the influence of CHCs on the quality of local services has been greatly reduced in many of the health authorities we visited in the course of our research. Perhaps the development of a more formal evaluative role for them might revive an important influence on the quality of services. Representatives of informed user groups can be involved in the quality improvement process itself, through membership of quality improvement groups, or participate in evaluation panels depending on their skills and interests.

Table 4.2   Analysing user involvement in the three modes of quality in Øvretveit's and our models

Modes of quality	Generic	Technical	Systemic
Client	Very high involvement possible both on individual basis and when represented by informed user groups	Only marginal as individual user but moderate when informed user group, particularly if specially constituted to involve outside experts	Moderate involvement possible when represented by informed user groups
Professional	Potentially very high but stereotype is of low involvement – e.g. 'arrogance' of consultants and different specialties denigrating one another	Obviously very high within specialties but requires a good deal of work to establish multi-professional systems – e.g. for audit	High within specialties; now also high at cross-functional level since doctors increasingly head up multiple specialty and multi-professional directorates
Management	Very high, particularly in setting the culture and context for maximizing the potential of all to contribute to service development	Low involvement but should be invited to attend and/or receive feedback on process and implications for strategic planning and resource management	Very high at all levels; however, the qualitative differences in nature of work at each level should be spelled out and associated with appropriate performance indicators

We have seen a range of important user-defined service improvements come out of the participation of outside representatives. In one case we heard about impressive results when community representatives were involved from the outset in the commissioning of a new community unit. In contrast, at another TQM location we observed the advanced stages of planning for a new unit based on the principles of patient-centred care where not a single outsider had been involved! It is significant that the level of understanding of the technicalities of TQM and its formal implementation were much higher at the site where there had been no involvement of users than at the location where users were involved in all the design stages. Clearly the more technical the TQM implementation, the more difficult it is for hospital staff to involve 'naive' users. It is essential, therefore, that training and other development is provided for those joining informed user groups. The training should cover TQM, evaluation and health systems, including issues of confidentiality.

The formation of informed user groups should also help to deal with problems associated with the commitment and reliability of participants because the growing knowledge and involvement resides in the group rather than just in individual members.

Figure 4.4   Involving users in evaluation at different levels

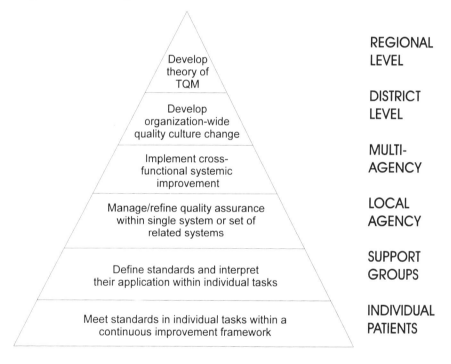

Involving users at higher levels in organizations

As we have discussed, an evaluation ought to consider what is going on in the higher levels of the organization, not just report on individual examples of service provision. We now go on to suggest that other outside interests should also be involved in evaluating the quality of work being undertaken at these higher levels. Figure 4.4 shows potential sources of outside involvement that we think might be appropriate at each level.

At the first level, individual patients and carers could be involved in planning their own care and providing feedback on their perceptions about quality of service. At the second level support groups and informed user groups would be involved in the process of setting and monitoring standards as well as ensuring that individual patients received appropriate quality of care.

Forward and backward mapping

As we discussed in Chapter 3, there is relatively little evidence of mapping of any kind in the NHS but those sites which had made the most elaborate arrangements for TQM were primarily involved in forward mapping. By this we mean that quality, and the structures and systems for managing quality improvement, were decided by senior management with little or no consultation with staff or external customers.

These decisions were then passed downwards and forwards through the organization ('cascaded' in management jargon) until they finally reached the customer. It was only then that some (limited) consultation took place, often on the basis of criteria defined by staff. Much was said about staff empowerment but this was beginning to take place at only a few of our sites. Similarly, what little involvement of patients and carers took place was normally confined to *post hoc* satisfaction questionnaires. It is relatively infrequent for patients, their carers and other organizations to have a say in the design of new systems or to set the criteria by which existing systems are evaluated.

In Figure 4.5 we have added the 'customer dimension'. The arrows describe the mainly forward and downward mapping of change. The strength of the process, indicated by arrow width, and the direction in which the arrows point, suggest the main traffic in information and involvement. This can be seen to be predominantly outwards in the form of dissemination of information rather than genuine involvement of outside groups in planning and evaluating services. There are changes taking place though, particularly at district level where the contracting process has considerably strengthened the hand of purchasers in setting quality standards and calling for information on the quality of services. Efforts need to be made to reverse this position at the other levels as well.

When to evaluate

Clearly a basic principle should be to get in and start an evaluation as soon as possible in the life of any organizational change because important decisions made early in the life of any project will be vital in understanding subsequent events. However, there are also some important decisions to be made about the style of evaluation before starting any data collection.

Formative or summative evaluation?

A basic distinction, which will later affect the way one goes about the

Figure 4.5 The forward-mapping process in NHS quality improvement

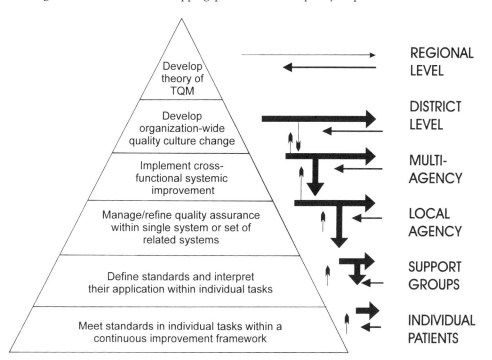

whole process, is whether to pursue a formative or summative evaluation (Scriven, 1967). In the context of TQM, a formative evaluation is one in which the evaluators work closely with programme managers and other organizational staff, regularly feeding back information from the evaluation and giving advice about the implications of the findings. The aim is to help staff in the organization to see more clearly what they are doing, achieving change through a better understanding.

The advantage of this style is that the programme managers get quick feedback on progress and can make changes to the implementation if it is not going too well. The disadvantage is that the evaluators will inevitably get drawn into the change process and may not be able to continue to report objectively at a later date.

A good example can be given from our evaluation of TQM in the NHS. We found at several sites that TQM skills' workshops which were organized as two-day events did not appear to be meeting the objectives for which they were set up. At other sites we found that a pattern of one afternoon session per week for six weeks with some project work in between seemed to work much better. This was also consistent with what we knew from research on the private sector. If we had been operating in a formative mode we could have recommended to the first group of sites that they switch to the second model. We could have been fairly confident (but by no means certain) that the training would have been improved.

However, suppose that we returned after six months and found that, contrary to our expectations, the situation was no better – would we have accurately reported the failure of training to meet its objectives, given that it was our idea to switch training models? What, subsequently, would have been our relationship with the programme managers, particularly in the event of a dispute about who was responsible for the lack of progress on training?

A summative evaluation, on the other hand, aims to provide an expert and objective assessment of the programme of change with as little 'contamination' as possible. The evaluators are normally from outside the organization. Although they may provide factual reports of their field-work at intervals, they confine their recommendations to a final report at the end of the evaluation. This is the style we adopted for the NHS evaluation.

Clearly a disadvantage of adopting a summative mode is that problems which become evident at an early stage in the evaluation may well not be put right, perhaps because the programme managers do not understand the implications of interim evaluation reports. This may cause an ethical dilemma for the evaluators and if the situation were serious enough they might have to move into a formative mode in order to bring the full implications to the attention of programme managers.

The choice of which style to adopt will depend on the purposes of the evaluation. In the case of the NHS TQM pilots, for example, we chose a summative mode because the Department of Health wanted an objective and critical appraisal of different models of TQM and their potential for improving the quality of public sector health care. There was considerable research-based consultancy support and literature on TQM already available to the NHS on TQM. Some sites took advantage of this and management consultants, in particular, played a significant formative role where they were asked to work with pilot sites on implementing TQM.

It is important to note that detailed measurement and evaluation are a central requirement of TQM and should therefore be a key feature of the design and implementation of any programme. As we have observed in Chapter 2, the nature of service delivery often makes data about both processes and outcomes transient, and continuous monitoring is therefore an important tool in getting quick feedback. The organization will also want to analyse data from the monitoring process and act on the implications as quickly as possible. This all suggests that a formative style is more appropriate for most organizational needs and best suits the role that internal evaluators would be expected to play.

However, the organization may well choose to commission an independent summative evaluation as an added source of critical feedback about progress. This might provide different and interesting insights into the change process. The additional confidence staff often have in the confidentiality provided by outside researchers may well mean that a more truthful picture will emerge.

Summary

Although there is a growing body of literature on the measurement of quality, there is less written about the issues of evaluation in health care. Evaluation requires one to make judgements about the results derived from measuring some aspect of health care and is a good deal more complex in this area than in most areas of the private sector where TQM had its origins. Evaluation in health care requires not only specific reference to personal and organizational values (by no means always clearly stated or agreed) but also consideration of the contrasting needs of a wide range of stakeholders.

Setting up and carrying out evaluations is often a resource-intensive and lengthy business and should not be entered into lightly. However, given that the comparative effects of different approaches to TQM in the NHS are not yet well understood we would advise prospective evaluators to set up as comprehensive an evaluation as can be afforded in terms of time and cost. It should, where possible, have the following features:

- *What to evaluate* should include a comprehensive set of criteria against which to evaluate progress. These should be based on the main requirements of TQM and include criteria generated by the organization, supplemented by others thought to be important by the evaluators. The criteria should encompass technical, systemic and generic issues. Framing criteria in terms of inputs, processes and outputs may be helpful. Criteria should include the conception of the TQM model, and progress on its implementation, as well as evidence of improvements in quality of service.
- *Where to evaluate* will depend on whether the evaluation is specifically targeted at one aspect of TQM or the organization, or whether it is a more comprehensive programme evaluation. For the latter, the evaluation should look at culture, structure, systems and process issues at all levels, not just at the interface between the operational base and service users.
- *Who should be involved in the evaluation* must take into account the different needs and perceptions of relevant stakeholders. This includes those working with the organization at each level, not just at the level of individual patients and carers. Stakeholders can make positive contributions to evaluating all modes of quality, not just generic quality for patients, technical quality for doctors and systemic quality for managers. Wherever possible, service users and other community members should be involved in designing and carrying out evaluations, in analysing the results and in planning changes to services.

- *When to measure* depends on the purposes of the evaluation, the budget, time-scale and skills of the evaluators. A formative style should be considered where rapid feedback about progress is required with supporting analysis and recommendations from the evaluators. A summative style should be considered when a more objective and considered evaluation is required and the programme managers want an evaluation which has been relatively uncontaminated by interim feedback to those who are being evaluated. TQM may best be evaluated by a combination of the two styles. Irrespective of style, as much time as possible must be allowed because of the long-term nature of TQM.

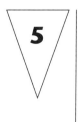

5 Learning from the NHS

Part I: Setting out the issues

We begin this chapter by outlining some of the key issues that face NHS sites in implementing TQM. We then discuss, in more detail, the results of our evaluation of TQM at a range of NHS units within eight health authorities from 1990 to 1993. We conclude the chapter with a summary of the main findings and implications for future TQM initiatives.

We noted in Chapter 2 that a considerable amount of quality improvement has gone on across the NHS for many years and this trend has accelerated more recently. Our own research revealed that all of the sites in our evaluation had a history of earlier, if mainly unsystematic, attempts at quality improvements. Indeed, it is important to note that at least two of the original eight district authorities in which we conducted research had begun TQM-style projects in some of their acute units prior to bidding for Department of Health funds.

Until the early 1980s, the choice of initiatives was very much a matter for district health authorities and what were later to become provider units. However, since the mid-1980s, all authorities and units have found themselves subjected to increasing pressure from the Department of Health to tackle what were seen at the centre as key areas for improvement – waiting times, facilities in public areas and provision of more choice to patients.

There were a number of reasons why the Department of Health chose TQM as a mechanism for generating change in the NHS. The main one was that key features of government reform in the NHS resonated strongly with some of the requirements of TQM. Table 5.1 suggests that three principles of TQM, in particular, were seen to be directly related to the main policy changes being sought by the government.

Table 5.1   A comparison of government reforms and the principles of TQM

NHS *changes*	TQM *principles*
Strengthening top management at each unit and involving doctors in management of services	Corporate approaches to planning, especially planning for quality – working towards common understandings and definitions of quality
Value for money	Continuous improvement through systematic measurement
Greater patient focus including more information, more choice and more involvement	Putting the customer at the centre of process improvement

Although the agenda moved on somewhat during the course of the evaluation, these factors have continued to be a central part of health reforms. By and large, however, our impression at the outset of the project was that a detailed understanding of the theories and concepts of TQM was limited to a small number of enthusiastic individuals at the centre. This meant that others at the centre, and at the TQM sites, played down some of the more controversial requirements of TQM which are held to be essential to its successful implementation. These included:

- the need to focus explicitly on the prevention of errors and the elimination of duplication or waste;
- the identification of internal customer–supplier chains which meant that doctors were essential to process improvement;
- compulsory TQM education and training for all staff.

A lack of preparedness to implement all these requirements was a key reason why TQM failed to take a hold at most of our sites.

Evaluating TQM at NHS sites

As we suggested in Chapters 3 and 4, there are some key features of orthodox models of TQM which one would expect to be put in place at any TQM site, even though the model of TQM being followed might lead to different methodologies. We therefore evaluated progress being made at each site in two ways. The first was against the objectives sites set for themselves (where these were specific enough for us to use as evaluative criteria) and also against key requirements of TQM – summarized here as *corporate approaches to quality, systematic measurement of quality*, and *customer-driven quality*. The main requirements in each area are discussed below.

Corporate approaches to quality

A major outcome of a successful TQM implementation would be increasingly well-developed corporate approaches to quality. Progress would be judged by the following criteria:

- the extent to which there is quality planning which is fully integrated with the normal business planning process;
- installation of structural changes to improve vertical and lateral accountability for quality;
- establishment of comprehensive performance review;
- the development of a senior management team which is actively committed to continuous quality improvement;
- an organization-wide quality planning system built on a common understanding of definitions of quality and the need for continuous improvement within a given model of TQM.

Achieving progress on corporate approaches was always going to be difficult in the NHS. As we described in Chapter 2, the NHS has a long tradition of consensus management between administrators and largely autonomous professional groups (see Table 2.4). Although there have also been strong hierarchies in place, as in the case of nursing, lateral relationships have been less well developed and definitions of quality have varied between different groups.

Review mechanisms have tended to focus on the quality of inputs and *post hoc* judgements about outputs. Developing good output measures has been difficult and focusing on systematic process improvement, particularly on 'designing in quality', has not been a feature of service development. Until recently, medical audit has been an exclusively doctor-driven process and the results have not normally been available to management for improvement purposes. Most arrangements for audit have been based on standard setting. This has proved to be a relatively static process concerning basic markers of good practice rather than a focus on continuous improvement as required by TQM.

Systematic measurement of quality

Under this heading one would expect to find the organization moving towards a model of 'management by fact'. At the start of TQM, the organization would be expected to assess how it stood on quality both in relation to its internal systems and processes and in terms of external customers' requirements (*diagnostics*). Increasingly one sees organizations, including NHS trusts, also measuring their performance against that of their competitors, particularly those who are seen to be leaders in their respective fields (*benchmarking*).[1] When we began our evaluation, the quality of information available in the NHS for general quality improvement purposes was variable. We expected it to be stronger in some of the technical and medical functions and weaker in administrative systems. Although this proved to be the case in most areas, there were some surprising exceptions.

Further, although the reliability and relevance of information might have been sufficient before TQM, it proved to be woefully inadequate to meet the needs of TQM-style continuous improvement. Take, for example, the process of discharging an elderly patient after an inpatient stay for an operation. Traditionally, the important information that was needed was whether or not the doctor had seen the patient, authorized the discharge and noted any requirements for post-stay care (for example, provision of take-home drugs). In our terms, this would principally be an issue of *technical* quality. However, one might want to know a lot more about the discharge process in terms of what we have called *systemic* and *generic* quality:

Technical quality
  Technical measures of recovery at the point of discharge. Correlation of level of recovery against different methods of post-operative medical treatment, dietary management, nursing skills, etc.
Systemic quality
  Quality of discharge process on the ward – for example, management of delay between authorization and actual discharge; quality of communication systems between other parties including relatives, etc.
  Quality of interface between ward systems and other internal systems – for example, theatres, X-ray, catering, pharmacy, patient welfare, etc.
  Quality of interface between ward systems and external systems – for example, the patient's GP, community services, social services, etc.
Generic quality
  Patient's views before, during and after discharge about the procedures. Quality of personal relationships between patient and staff including standards of courtesy, dignity, privacy, confidentiality, etc.

Personal versus departmental performance
Another key area of data concerns personal rather than departmental performance. Under TQM one would require personal performance measures to be developed which reinforce the importance of the principles of TQM. Prior to TQM, there were few measures of personal performance in place for most groups of staff. Indeed, quality criteria were not very explicit or related to personal behaviour, apart from a few obvious areas such as pathology where there was considerable individual attention to the pursuit of well-defined quality criteria.

The main instrument of performance measurement was the individual performance review (IPR) but, as we discuss in more detail later, few staff thought that this set personal quality improvement objectives or that the system actually influenced their day-to-day behaviour. Where standards had been developed and put in place, we found little evidence that these were either tied to, or being used to measure, personal performance.

Customer-driven satisfaction

Most NHS staff will claim that they are motivated principally by the desire to help others and that patient satisfaction is the driving force behind their work. However, our research found that before TQM started most staff were driven principally by professional and technical definitions of quality which were, at best, only tenuously related to consumer-based definitions of quality (consumers here are taken to be patients, their relatives and other carers and, more generally, the communities in which the sites were located). Professionals assumed, rather than made explicit, an altruistic concern for their patients.

In our interviews, medical and nursing staff stated that, in the past, quality would have been seen in terms of technical and medical outcomes rather than more holistic concerns with patient satisfaction. This view was also prevalent in areas such as catering and domestic services. Even where nursing standards had been defined these appeared, by and large, to have been based on professional views of patient need rather than asking the patients what they wanted.

There were, however, some exceptions to these specialist views of patient need – for example, in maternity and psychiatric services where there had been an increasing recognition of the need to build the views of patients and relatives into the care planning process. Hospital services for children were also likely to have taken a broad perspective on patient need before TQM started. In some specialties, active and sophisticated interest groups contributed to the widening of perspectives.

One of the most significant findings of our evaluation was the extent to which there had been a general shift from professional and technical definitions of quality towards 'customer-oriented' views of quality. Of course, many factors have contributed to this shift – the purchaser–provider split, contracting, the move to trust status, the Patient's Charter, compulsory competitive tendering, and quality assurance. However, the shift was stronger at our NHS TQM sites than at those implementing other forms of quality improvement, suggesting that TQM had had a significant effect in its own right.

We should distinguish here between a focus on customers and actually empowering them. Many NHS districts and provider units now provide a vastly improved information service to patients, carers, GPs and other customers. Improved provision of information was a significant development at our TQM demonstration sites. However, this is a long way from empowerment. Much of the information had still been produced without consultation with patients and sometimes failed to tackle issues that were of importance to them. Further, additional general information did not always go with improved choice, or with transparent management – both of which could be considered to be essential features of TQM in a public sector setting (see, for example, Pfeffer and Coote, 1991).

We look now in more detail at some of the significant results of implementing TQM at the NHS demonstration sites in our sample.

Part II: Some key results from our evaluation of TQM

The project began with fieldwork in eight districts – Bolton, Doncaster, Liverpool, Merton and Sutton, South East Stafford, Trafford, Winchester and Worthing. The principal means of data gathering was a series of semi-structured, one-to-one confidential interviews of around an hour's duration with a wide range of staff from all levels at each site. Because we interviewed in three successive years, we were able to speak to many staff on more than one occasion. In all, we interviewed 569 people at both district and provider-unit level in a range of NHS demonstration sites during the summers of 1991, 1992 and 1993.

Seventy-seven per cent of those interviewed in 1991 were interviewed again in 1992, and 60% of those interviewed in 1992 were interviewed again in 1993. A further 177 staff were interviewed at four NHS comparator sites which were not implementing TQM (although they were implementing a number of other quality initiatives); 67% of the sample were interviewed in both years. Appendix IV shows the roles and levels of staff interviewed at the TQM and non-TQM sites.

In addition, we interviewed 104 staff in two commercial organizations, Thames Water Utilities and Post Office Counters, in the spring of 1992 and 1993, with some 55% being interviewed in both years. At the start of the evaluation, Post Office Counters was in the early stages of introducing an orthodox TQM initiative called 'Customer First'. This was being piloted in headquarters departments and in three divisions. Thames Water was following a more evolutionary approach, trying out three different quality initiatives – an internal quality award programme ('Thames Quality Awards'), BS 5750 in the engineering function, and two TQM pilots at sewage treatment works (see Chapter 6 for a full discussion of the implications of our findings). We also analysed a considerable amount of documentary material from each site and attended a number of key meetings and training events.

Although the original intention was to work at one location in each of eight health districts, the shift to trust status for many units meant a considerable increase in variation of approaches to TQM. To ensure breadth of coverage we initially interviewed at 31 different hospitals or community services in the TQM NHS districts in the first year, and followed up 25 of these locations over the next three years. Between them these eight authorities offered a reasonable range of locations and distribution of facilities. Over the course of the project all but two units applied for and secured trust status. The sample included a range of large acute units, including one teaching hospital, smaller community hospitals, and several community services.

Quality states prior to the start of TQM

For the most part, the decision at the NHS sites to install TQM or QA was not problem-led. Where there were concerns about quality, these were typical of large complex organizations delivering a wide range of services in the public sector. The factors that triggered a decision to implement TQM at a local level varied. For example, those units that were applying for trust status were aware that bids were unlikely to be successful if arrangements for quality assurance were not given a high profile. Other factors were also influential. The appointment of a new district general manager or chief executive with an interest in some of the principles of TQM could start an initiative. Other triggers that proved influential included:

- a desire to integrate professionals and managers within the general management structure;
- the need to integrate the diverse cultures of hospitals which were now being merged into larger units;
- a desire to change the culture of residential services;
- the need to find further ways to save money;
- a totally pragmatic decision not to turn down money that the Department was making available;
- the need to provide coherent integration of a wide range of existing and new initiatives including the Resource Management Initiative (RMI), medical audit, nursing audit, the work of quality circles and the Personalizing the Service Initiative (PSI), the purchaser–provider split, compulsory competitive tendering, introduction of standard setting, devolved budgets, and the Patient's Charter.

The issue of resources and forms of quality improvement

There was widespread, but not unanimous, feeling that resources were inadequate to provide the level of service respondents felt they should be giving. Compulsory competitive tendering and cost improvement exercises were squeezing resources and many respondents considered that staff morale was low. Despite financial restrictions, increasingly heavy workloads, and statements about low morale, staff continued to try out many new ideas for service improvement.

The actual number of projects varied from site to site. However, the impression we formed from respondents' descriptions during our first round of fieldwork in 1991 was that pre-TQM initiatives were often one-off attempts to improve the quality of an individual process (or part of a process) rather than as part of a full quality assurance programme. Quite a few examples we were given were projects that individuals were carrying out as part of further education or professional qualifications. Most of the examples we heard were:

- initiatives driven by interested individuals, often ploughing a lonely furrow;
- limited to the internal workings of a single department;
- projects where staff felt that they were not supported by management through recognition or provision of resources;
- projects which were not normally integrated with other initiatives;
- not integrated with the general strategic thrust of the unit or service.

Staff attitudes

Prior to the start of TQM many of our interviewees reported that there was an over-reliance on the professional expert and medical models of patient care rather than a more holistic understanding of *total* patient care. Thus, insufficient attention was seen as being paid to the patients' emotional and non-medical needs. Patients were often treated as passive by nurses and doctors who were more task-oriented than patient-oriented. Nurses, both front-line and managers, referred many times to what they called 'the arrogance of consultants' and/or to the unwarranted certainty they displayed towards patients and other staff (cf. Schön, 1983; Steffen, 1988).

Similarly, it was put to us that systems and staff sometimes appeared to be geared more to meeting staff needs than those of patients. Examples included wider choice and better quality of food for staff than that destined for patients; unnecessary restrictions on visiting hours; lack of parking for visitors and staff parking in visitors' bays; patients on wards still woken very early in the morning; and consultants who arrived late for clinics, or who held them at times inconvenient to the users.

Communication – internal and external

Problems with internal communication were high on the agenda. The reasons given were many and varied. Communications between different professional groups were strained. It was said that there was a lack of multi-disciplinary working, both within hospitals and between hospitals and other services. Systemic problems also arose which led to a lack of coordination between internal customers. Common examples were between doctors and the therapy professions, X-ray and the wards; between wards and functions such as catering and laundry; and between finance or personnel and their internal customers. One of the important advances made by TQM was improved communication between some of these groups. For example, we received enthusiastic accounts of improvements between teams of people working at the operational level in finance and personnel at one site and between wards and catering at another.

Design of new systems

It was said that new organizational structures were designed and implemented with little consultation or with inadequate information – something that still tended to happen after TQM was implemented. The fact that some departments were already beginning to make changes at the outset of TQM could lead to problems when other departments in the same process had not moved as far. For example, mothers-to-be in one maternity hospital found that some ante-natal processes were prepared to include the father and other relatives in discussions about procedures, but just down the corridor, in the ultrasound unit, even fathers were excluded.

Concepts of quality prior to the start of TQM

There were few significant differences in concepts of quality between the TQM locations and the comparison sites which had non-TQM quality initiatives in place. Taking all the sites together, the scatter of assumptions about the meaning of quality was wide. They included: speed of response and waiting times; staff appearance; the public image of the hospital; continuous improvement; monitoring the speed at which complaints were dealt with; individualized patient care; good working environment; good resource management; safety; good medical environment and clinical standards; and supervision of learners.

Having said this, some of these concepts were mentioned more often than others. For example, the issues of errors and waste were not particularly high on the NHS agenda – certainly not as high as they were at the two commercial companies. Similarly, respondents in the commercial companies were more critical of staff attitudes and behaviour than their counterparts in the NHS. NHS staff felt that they already had an overriding concern with patients' interests, though many believed there was an over-reliance on a professional expert and medical model.

Although definitions of quality were somewhat uncertain and varied, most staff groups had their own standards. These were derived from a combination of professional training and guidance, legal prescription, national and local criteria imposed by sources outside the organization, and standards laid down by the organizations themselves. These were apparent in job descriptions, IPR objectives, union agreements, and standards of professional practice.

For example, in one hospital, porters had their 'do's and don'ts' about smoking in areas to which the public had access; pathologists had strict quality control procedures for tests based on national norms; finance followed financial rules and prescribed accounting practice; medical engineering complied with BS 5724; catering had to meet national hygiene regulations, and medical staff followed ethical and practical guidelines provided by their colleges and national committees.

A number of the interviewees recognized that the standards existing before TQM were different from definitions of quality under TQM. For example, a pathologist noted that the specialist focus on technical excellence should be broadened to include issues of customer satisfaction (i.e. satisfaction with the service given to GPs, hospital doctors and patients).

Some of the nurse managers and nurses saw that setting nursing standards did not necessarily meet the principles of continuous improvement under TQM. Other interviewees saw the need to integrate changes in organization, structure and systems, in order to widen definitions of quality to include the users' views. Some further concepts which were held to be common prior to the start of the projects are discussed below.

There was a prevalent view among interviewees that, prior to the introduction of TQM, definitions of quality would have been individualistic or particular to different professional groups. These, in turn, would have depended on the professional training and experience. Thus concepts of quality in obstetrics, psychiatry, medical engineering and linen services would have been quite different.

This would be so not only in their technical core, as might be expected, but also in such dimensions as relationships with patients, where one might expect a more generic approach. Even within these different areas there would have been difficulties in getting common agreement about definitions of quality. The specialist base would not be eroded by TQM but would be complemented by generic and systemic concepts of quality.

Changes in definitions and concepts of quality during the evaluation

An important requirement under TQM is that there should be a progressive convergence towards common definitions of quality. In the commercial sector, for example, all staff would be encouraged to follow a single definition of quality. There were marked differences between the NHS sites in this respect. At one extreme there was almost no movement at all towards a single organizational definition at two of the sites, through to marked movements towards common definitions at two others. The rest of the sites lay somewhere in between. Analysis of differences showed that the amount of movement could be accounted for by four key variables:

Training: Where a significant amount of training had taken place *and* the widespread dissemination of a particular definition of quality was part of that training, then there was less variation in definitions of quality.

Management consultants: Where sites had employed firms of management consultants, definitions used by the consultants tended to have taken a firm hold. Interestingly, at one site, this was so even though the services of the management consultants had been dispensed with after the initial diagnostic phase and little further training had taken place.

Organizational definitions: Where little or no attempt had been made to propose and disseminate an organizational definition, we found more variability in personal definitions. It was clear that proposing an organizational definition on its own was not sufficient for it to take hold. This only occurred if that definition was disseminated through training events and through other mechanisms – for example, separate quality structures, meetings and projects and internal documentation, including newsletters.

Following a distinct TQM approach: Where sites which were following a particular TQM model – for example, Crosby – or a model developed by management consultants, respondents were much more likely to produce common definitions based on the model that the site was following.

It is important to note that even at sites where there had been less progress towards a definition proposed by the organization, we could detect important shifts towards the basic philosophy of TQM. The main themes were:

* A shift from focusing on inputs – for example, a lack of resources *per se* – to a concern with outputs and optimum use of resources.
* A shift from focusing on environmental improvement to process improvement with more of a customer orientation (quite common); and a move to process improvement with a view to reducing waste and error (still quite rare).
* A shift from exclusive dependence on technical/professional views of quality to more holistic patient-centred ones. This grew quite rapidly in the first year of the project and had become clearer and more sustained by 1993. It should be said, however, that considerable variation still existed within individual sites.

There had been a progressive move towards the general concept of internal customers, particularly at those sites following a structured TQM approach. The concept was strongest at those sites where they were following a specific form of TQM and where the idea was promoted in training. In contrast, the principle of internal customer–supplier chains had really only begun to appear in one or two departments at a few sites. Typically it had been taken up in some clinical support services (for example, pharmacy) and non-clinical support services (finance or personnel).

Level of understanding of TQM concepts

Although there were differences between the sites in terms of respondents' understanding of the concepts of TQM, the extent to which they felt that they had a better understanding was, not surprisingly, correlated with the amount of training they had had in their own particular schemes. We reported in 1992 that at three sites where there had been little or no training, as many as one-third of respondents said they had little or no understanding of their schemes at all. By and large this was still the case after a further year of TQM, at least up until the summer of 1993. Those respondents who had continued to get further training in 1992 and 1993 reported an increase in understanding of and commitment to TQM.

Even where interviewees had had no further training, but had been involved in quality improvement projects, they also gave positive views of TQM and stated they had a better understanding of TQM implementation because of continued involvement. It was also noteworthy that those senior

managers who spoke with most conviction about particular approaches to
TQM were those who had visited the USA to look at TQM in the health
sector, or who had otherwise been closely involved with TQM management consultants since the start of their projects. Staff who had had no
training and no involvement in improvement projects had much more
negative views of TQM. We also found this to be the case in the commercial organizations in our sample, and it emphasizes the importance of early
involvement of staff in both training and quality improvement projects.

Corporate approaches to quality improvement

Pre-TQM diagnostics
As discussed above, TQM requires the implementation of an organization-
wide quality planning system built on a common understanding of definitions of quality and the need for continuous improvement within a given
model of TQM. This, in turn, suggests that the organization has carried
out a thorough diagnosis of its starting position – both for planning purposes and also to be able to measure progress at some future point.

   We found that few of the NHS sites carried out any diagnostics or
benchmarking at the outset of the TQM initiatives. One or two undertook
staff surveys, while others had data which had been collected from spo-
radic patient surveys. Elsewhere specific services had carried out their own
studies for reasons unconnected to TQM. For example, in one authority,
sophisticated epidemiological studies and patient satisfaction surveys had
been carried out over the previous four years in public dental health.

   Generally speaking, we formed the opinion that dental services were in
advance of other services – in many respects they were already operating
within a basic TQM framework. Little diagnostic work had been undertaken at the non-TQM NHS sites either, although a site which was en-
gaged in a King's Fund organizational audit had set up an organizational
development group which had undertaken some staff attitude survey work.
A pharmaceutical service at the same hospital had carried out an elaborate
interview-based survey programme of its internal customers.

   Only one TQM site had carried out a comprehensive diagnostic exercise. It was undertaken by management consultants as part of setting up
TQM. It included a thorough staff attitude survey, a survey of 110 GPs,
interviews with patients and other interested parties with experience of the
services, a more general survey of residents in the area and a confidential
study of medical audit. Taken together, the results helped senior management to identify the gaps between what they saw as the goals and objectives for the future and what they were told by key stakeholders. It is
significant that this organization had already perceived that it was under
threat from its larger neighbours and wanted to develop a range of services
which were explicitly designed to be locally based and directly matched to
the needs of local users.

The planning process

Sites that bid for Department of Health money had to submit proposals which included details of proposed planning processes. The amount of detail in the bids varied, and in some cases bids amounted to little more than a bare outline. Progress reports provided by the sites a year after their start showed little evidence of well-organized monitoring and evaluation. All the TQM-funded projects had issued mission statements with varying degrees of specificity.

The terms under which successful proposals were accepted illuminate the Department of Health's thinking at that time. It was clear that the Department was content to allow sites to develop their own approaches to TQM. It was hoped that this would encourage sites to 'own' their own approaches and to allow a range of different approaches to be tested. It can be seen that there is a marked contrast between this approach and the one the Department took to the Patient's Charter. The Charter was centrally driven, explicit in context and framed around centrally set objectives and time-scales. There was also a requirement for continuous monitoring of both the implementation of the Charter and a number of key standards.

Only three sites involved more junior staff in work on mission and philosophy statements and it was significant that all these projects were led by management consultants. Only four of the original eight authorities turned mission statements into measurable objectives as part of their TQM initiative, although the introduction of business planning at all sites later increased the specificity of the objectives set. Indeed, the pressures of the purchaser–provider split and the resulting contracting process had been more influential on corporate planning than TQM. Departments which were not yet developing specific contracts for internal or external customers had weaker quality objectives than departments which were subject to strong purchaser pressure, although all of them were theoretically subject to TQM.

At the non-TQM NHS sites, each year of the evaluation showed increased corporate planning activity, although it is significant that the quality dimension was markedly weaker than at TQM sites which were making most progress. A clear difficulty for the non-TQM sites was the fact that there were so many different initiatives being driven by different departments and functions. The lack of an organization-wide quality steering group and quality structure within directorates made it more difficult to integrate these different initiatives.

Structural issues

All models of TQM stress the need for changes to the organizational structure in order to encourage and support the quality improvement process. However, tensions exist between structures which emphasize the role of line managers in quality and those which result in a complete shadow structure for implementing TQM. TQM argues for structures which:

- reduce barriers between different functions and groups;
- provide explicit vertical and lateral accountability for quality throughout the organization, including closer cooperation between management and professional roles;
- support improved multi-disciplinary and multi-functional working towards continuous quality improvement.

Structuring for quality at the NHS sites should be seen against a background of continuous organizational change since 1990. Almost all the sites had moved progressively towards implementation of clinical directorates. This, combined with work on trust applications, had slowed down the implementation of structures for handling TQM implementation. While most of the TQM sites had managed to put a unit-wide quality steering group in place and appoint a quality manager, there was no progress at all at two sites below quality steering group level. Elsewhere only two sites had established quality improvement teams across a substantial number of units.

All the TQM sites had established other groups for tackling quality improvement outside TQM. Many of these groups were operating on different assumptions about quality, using different methodologies and either duplicating, or otherwise getting in the way of, the work of other groups. They included quality circles, quality action teams, problem-solving teams, King's Fund audit groups, BS 5750 groups, standard-setting groups, and a wide range of committees, divisional meetings and specialty meetings. Only one of the TQM sites had got to grips with integrating new initiatives within a common TQM framework.

The gap between medical audit and broader forms of clinical audit was a salient feature at most sites. The gulf between doctors and the rest of the staff was well illustrated by the fact that at three hospitals the TQM managers had no idea of how much money was provided for medical audit at the site, did not know how it was spent and did not know what was being achieved through the use of the money. While there were obvious difficulties because of the issue of confidentiality, many staff expressed criticism of, and frustration with, the current relationship between medical audit and other modes of audit.

There was general support for a shift from funding of medical audit to funding of clinical or process-based audit. This support included a number of medical consultants who were themselves critical of the medical audit system. Two chief executives also felt that medical audit needed to become a source of information feeding into decisions of planning and resource allocation. However, some doctors were concerned that unless the money continued to be ring-fenced, chief executives might be tempted to use the money for non-audit purposes.

Provision of resources for NHS TQM implementation

We consider the resourcing of TQM at the NHS sites under two separate headings – education and training, and general funding of TQM. Resourcing, generally, was one of the areas which showed the biggest differences within the NHS TQM sample and between the NHS, generally, and the commercial companies.

Education and training for quality improvement

The resources made available for TQM implementation should provide for sufficient education and training and support to equip all staff with the commitment and skills to implement customer-driven continuous improvement. The word 'education' is used to emphasize the attitudinal and cultural changes required, while training usually refers to providing specific tools and techniques.

Given how dependent TQM is on effective education and training to lead change, it is surprising how little had been conducted at many of the NHS sites. Several locations began with two-hour programmes of 'awareness raising' to large numbers of staff. At one site they completed sessions for 1,900 out of a target group of 2,500 staff. This was accomplished by eight pairs of trainers in some 90 sessions over seven weeks.

However, as at most sites that started in this way, there was no follow-up with more extended tools and techniques training. After awareness sessions (where they took place), training was normally carried out on a top-down basis. Thus, typically, there were workshops for senior management teams which lasted from one to three days. These were often facilitated by external consultants. In several instances these workshops were used to develop the organization's mission statement, its values and objectives.

An important variation was developed at one of the sites. This was a detailed 'Introducing Quality Management' training pack, which provided for anything from half a day's awareness raising to an intensive two-day workshop on quality. This pack was subsequently successfully sold to a large number of other authorities. Another approach was to hold one- or two-day customer awareness training events. These were often hosted away from the workplace, run by professional facilitators from training organizations, and designed to raise awareness of the importance of the ultimate customer or end user.

The sites which followed Crosby or Crosby-like programmes had altogether more comprehensive training. Internal trainers were trained by external consultants and then combinations of trainers and managers conducted weekly workshops of around two hours' duration for multidisciplinary and multi-level groups of staff. These ran for between eight and ten weeks. Further, shorter programmes were then run in the workplace as part of training for front-line teams. The site with the widest coverage had trained 550 managers, supervisors and senior professionals including 40 medical consultants. More than 2,500 staff from a total of 3,000 had been trained in a work-group setting. This level of training was far in excess of any other site.

This site had also encouraged more than 30 consultants to attend training.

However, other sites had not reached anything like this figure – it was typically under 5% for consultants and other senior medical staff, and under 1% for junior doctors. Although time and money were frequently cited as reasons why doctors had not attended training, it was clear that the general unwillingness of many doctors to accept the underlying principles of TQM was at the heart of their non-attendance. It seemed unlikely that this would improve at most sites unless better ways could be found to operationalize the philosophy of TQM so as to encompass medical and professional viewpoints. This issue is taken up further in Chapter 8.

A specific problem about multi-disciplinary and multi-level courses became apparent at an early stage and still requires careful consideration. This concerned the disparity in levels of skills among participants. The courses were greatly valued for the opportunity they gave front-line staff to meet colleagues in other departments and also more senior staff in a wide range of different functions. This aspect appeared to work well as far as awareness raising was concerned, but not when participants began to tackle some of the process improvement tools and techniques.

It was quite likely that on a course one would find some scientists, research staff and doctors with a developed understanding of research methodology and descriptive statistics mixed with staff who had had little opportunity or experience in these areas. A significant proportion of the latter group felt uncomfortable with the technical aspects of measurement and analysis and were often intimidated by the skills displayed by professional staff. Trainers and managers had tried to take this into account by running the courses at a fairly basic level but this, in turn, had raised considerable criticism from staff who were already familiar with basic data collection and analysis techniques. In some cases the skills gap proved too wide to bridge.

We feel, however, that general awareness raising events which are confined to discussions about the basic principles of TQM and which are designed to improve communication within and between departments, are quite capable of being run on a multi-disciplinary and multi-level basis. This kind of event could be followed by specific tools and techniques training for uni-disciplinary groups of staff where the material could be directly related to the experience of the participants (see Figure 5.1).

They could then be involved in tackling process improvement issues in their own areas of work. Once staff were trained and working in quality improvement groups or teams, there might be some further opportunity to facilitate multi-disciplinary work by 'training' the actual teams themselves or running cross-functional process improvement exercises.

The training provided at the NHS TQM sites compares unfavourably with the altogether more substantial training undertaken at the commercial locations. At Thames Water 48 facilitators had been appointed and trained on a programme lasting two and a half days. This was followed by further personal development over a 12-month period leading to validation as internal auditors. Training at the pilot TQM sites at Thames had

Figure 5.1 Uni- and multi-disciplinary arrangements for training

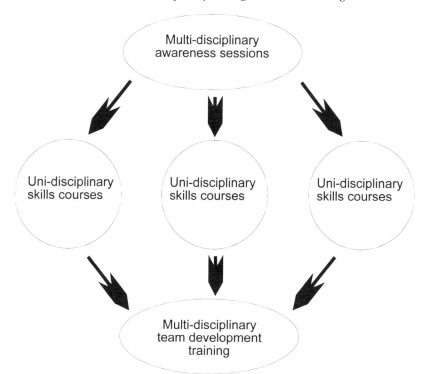

provided managers with a one-day general awareness event, while team leaders of process improvement teams received an additional two days on facilitation and teamwork skills and three days on statistical process control.

The quality support managers at Post Office Counters had a six-week training course run by management consultants with up to three weeks' further training over the following three years. The senior and middle management course was a 'five-day plus five-day' course. Junior staff had a one-day general introduction followed by six modules of training over a period of six months. These modules were interspersed by practical training through quality improvement projects.

General funding of TQM
At the outset of the project our intention was to analyse, in some detail, the costs of implementing TQM. We also expected to be able to collect some data on the savings to be made from its implementation. In the event, this proved to be considerably more difficult than expected. This was primarily because most sites had not kept accurate records of TQM expenditure, and devolution of budgets meant that expenditure was fragmented and less easy to trace. There were many sources of funds, for

Table 5.2   Quality improvement funding for two contrasting NHS sites

Site 1

Resources	Costs (£000s)
External management consultancy	20–50
Two full-time quality facilitators	50
Part-time quality assistant posts	35
Non-medical audit projects	40
Costs of medical audit	120
Customer care/standard-setting training	10
Total	275–305

Site 2

Resources	Costs (£000s)
Medical audit	80
Quality department salaries	80
Management consultancy from the region	50
Charter fellowship research on cancelled operations	10
Management competence research (regional funding)	5
District Health Authority for information to patients	15
Multi-disciplinary audit of therapy profession	10
Total	250

quality improvement activity of different kinds. Often only relatively small amounts were provided, although together these would constitute a considerable sum. Table 5.2 shows how two sites came up with roughly similar figures, but using completely different criteria.

At site 1 the cost of training is comparatively low, and at site 2 it is not shown. However, if a site were to engage in comprehensive training, costs could rise substantially, particularly if management consultants were employed. The demonstration site which had used consultants estimated it had spent around £40,000 on pre-planning for training and a further £100,000 on training the trainers and on material for courses over the first three years.

The figures for site 2 appear substantial, but they are only around a third of what Post Office Counters and Thames Water Utilities (our two comparator sites) spent on TQM for similar numbers of staff. Post Office Counters' expenditure on TQM averaged £1 million a year for the first three years for three pilot districts (roughly equivalent in workforce terms to a small provider unit). Thames Water's estimates were roughly comparable with those of Post Office Counters when calculated on a per-capita basis. The main differences were in the amount spent on training and on internal and external surveys. Post Office Counters, in particular, spent substantial amounts of money on identifying what customers (post office users and major agency customers) wanted from the services that they provided.

The inclusion of medical audit money in the NHS figures disguises the small amount available to quality departments for implementing TQM. Furthermore, funding had been reduced progressively since 1990 at several sites. For example, at one site in 1992 the Quality Manager was fighting to secure a budget of only £9,000 to provide some much needed training for key staff. Two other large multiple-site acute units were expected to implement TQM on budgets of under £60,000 per year, and it was not unusual to find only one or two quality facilitators for sites of around 5,000 staff. One community service, which had made considerable advances in implementing TQM, had had to reduce work-group training sessions, which were previously of three hours' duration for around 14 staff, to sessions of only one hour for larger numbers.

It is important to note that all the sites from which we were able to secure some details about costs of TQM exceeded the amounts they were given by the Department of Health for TQM funding. Originally, seven out of the eight authorities had been funded for two years and one for one year. Of the former, funding over the two years ranged from between £45,000 and £90,000 (including support from the region where this had been forthcoming). The eighth authority had received £20,000 for its first year.

Even these figures may be misleading since in some places all the money went to just one location, whereas in other cases it was split between several provider units. Other than absolute size, what proved to be important about this money was that it was relatively firmly ring-fenced for quality improvement purposes. It at least entailed the funding of one or more quality managers or facilitators, specifically mandated to implement TQM.

When the Department of Health funding ran out, continuation at most sites depended almost entirely on the attitude of the Unit General Manager or chief executive. Until 1992 all sites managed to continue funding at least the central post of quality manager. However, for reasons which were not entirely clear, and may not have been financial, two sites had made the quality managers redundant and showed no signs of replacing them. Our general impression was that front-line staff read this as an indication that TQM was being put 'on the back burner', if not being abandoned altogether.

Savings made by TQM

Proponents of TQM in the commercial sector claim that considerable savings can be made by introducing TQM. The literature talks expansively about savings of 15–40% through reductions in error and waste (see, for example, Atkinson, 1990). There is some evidence that similar savings are possible in the public sector. A report of one study of a ward for the elderly in an acute unit showed that 17% of costs could be saved by attention to six or seven key areas (Joss, 1995). Similar studies in acute units and community services by Koch (1993) showed average savings of 5–15% of budget in many service areas with some figures as high as 38% (for example, in radiology and some community services). Most of the NHS sites we visited had not looked at the cost of poor quality in this way.

However, there are many examples of savings which point to what might be possible when all processes in a particular department are subject to scrutiny. Typical examples include a pharmacy department which made an annual saving of £13,000 following a two-month review of stock held in dispensaries, and an outpatients department that made savings of £3,000 a year by reducing the amount of stock carried. This was achieved by applying standard materials management techniques. In another hospital a study of wastage of food, previously running at £1,000 per month, had been cut by 50% in nine months.

Several other process improvement projects have also made spectacular savings, although accurate figures are not available. Two services, for example, both found that wheelchairs and walking aids were disappearing at unacceptable rates. The imposition of a £10 deposit on equipment had dramatically reduced losses. In one hospital this had been supported by allowing people to return equipment to doctors' surgeries, health centres and other locations, rather than returning it to the hospital. Initially there had been widespread reaction against the idea of putting deposits on wheelchairs, but none had disappeared since and it had now become accepted policy. These examples point to the kinds of saving that could be made. Our experience suggests that savings of 10–20% on departmental budgets across a complete unit would be achievable, though not all of this could be recovered in the first year of a TQM programme.

We should emphasize again that many of these projects were being designed and implemented by highly committed and competent staff on an individual basis and therefore it was rare to find comprehensive activity going on across more than one or two departments in any unit we visited. The lack of training in specific process improvement tools and techniques in most units meant that most staff, even if they were committed to TQM, did not have the skills to implement continuous improvement in their own processes. In addition, all but three of the sample had yet to implement quality improvement groups or teams at departmental level, other than in one or two lead departments. This again meant that there was no mechanism for encouraging a wider group of staff to get involved in quality initiatives.

Systematic measurement

Systematic measurement is a key feature of TQM. We looked at three areas – information provision, monitoring and evaluation, and process improvement.

Information provision

Successful implementation of TQM depends on the availability of high-quality information for process improvement purposes. It is referred to in much of the literature as 'management by fact'. Information is of high quality if it is accurate, timely and relevant to the needs of internal and external customers.

Most of the NHS sites, TQM and non-TQM, started in a relatively poor position in this respect. There was a fair amount of information available already, but this was not always as reliable as TQM would require and rarely in a form suitable for process improvement. Most sites were carrying out some form of patient satisfaction survey in a number of areas, and there was a wealth of financial performance information also available, albeit not necessarily in a form helpful to potential users. A number of other initiatives were either calling for, or actually providing, new levels and new kinds of information. The waiting list and outpatients initiatives required the introduction of better appointment systems, and elsewhere the Patient's Charter and contracting began to specify standards which had to be monitored on a regular basis.

In addition, the Resource Management Initiative (RMI) was beginning to influence clinicians, principally towards basing decision-making about resource allocation on the basis of more reliable information. Further, medical, clinical and nursing audit arrangements were also beginning to produce data on both processes and outcomes in ways which were more systematic than had been the case before. Now, three years on, a plethora of different systems, both manual and computer-based, has been introduced. Some of the systems mentioned were MONITOR, THEATREMAN, ITUMAN, CRESCENDO, PATSAT, QAID and QARX. In addition, we came across many more examples including purpose-developed systems for individual units as far apart as X-ray, catering and some community services.

There is little doubt that there have been major improvements in the information now available for process improvement purposes. However, even with imaginative use, it is often the case that information being provided by the systems described above will never be able to meet most of the needs of quality improvement groups or teams. The information continued to suffer from three weaknesses.

First, it was rare to find detailed information about small stages of a process which was essential for TQM – for example, the time taken to repair a piece of equipment, or the number of times a doctor's remarks on a request for an analysis of blood were illegible.

Second, information about processes was often held on different information systems and could not provide essential data about a complete process – for example, the time taken to complete all the stages of getting a patient from a ward to X-ray and back. This meant quality improvement groups had to collect the data for themselves. Since few sites had provided them with training in data collection techniques (see the discussion of training provision, above), proper detailed data collection either never took place or was only partially completed. Continuous monitoring was rarely feasible.

Third, data were still on the crude side and based, in the main, on over-simplified quantitative measures such as waiting times or waiting lists. Connections made between complicated relationships – for example, those between activity, skills mix and patient dependency – were poor.

By and large there were few quality improvement groups or directorate quality staff with the requisite skills to design and carry out effective analysis of anything more than the simplest of systems. Where there were exceptions to this, it was because there were one or two key individuals who had picked up their research skills in the course of doing external qualifications or because they had, in the past, worked in a research capacity. It was rare to find that anything other than basic training on tools and techniques for data analysis had been provided to members of quality improvement groups. More often than not, even quality facilitators had little or no training.

Measures of personal performance

Much of the literature on TQM suggests that the long-term success of this approach depends on being able to embed the principles of TQM into the very fabric of the organization. This would include reorienting the processes by which the performance of individuals and their sections or departments are monitored. This is seen to be particularly important in management roles, in support services and in other areas where there is limited contact with external customers. Thus, under orthodox TQM, all members of an organization (and collectively each department) would identify who their internal and external customers were and performance would then be monitored on the basis of the extent to which each person or the department met or exceeded these customers' requirements.

As far as individual review was concerned, we distinguished between clinical performance and the more general or managerial aspects of people's roles. Clinical performance had to comply with national or local guidelines and protocols of professional bodies. These were not explicitly linked to customers' requirements, other than the requirements of regulatory or auditing bodies.

Personal standards were most likely to be found in front-line roles where there was strong technical content to the work – for example, in pathology, pharmacy and some nursing roles. We found personal standards where results could be traced back to individuals because they had direct, and definable, contact with users. However, the standards were still likely to have been set by managers or professional staff based on technical and professional criteria rather than on internal or external users' expressed requirements.

Many of the non-medical staff we interviewed were subject to individual performance review. However, our observations were that IPR was insufficient to serve as a reinforcing mechanism for implementing TQM. Some of the weaknesses were:

- objectives under IPR generally referred to the performance of groups of staff rather than personal performance targets;
- IPRs were usually an annual event and less than 5% of respondents felt that the process significantly affected their day-to-day behaviour;
- an appreciable number of staff had not had an IPR for as long as three or four years, while others had been in their roles for nearly a year before any objective-setting exercise took place;
- IPRs for managers set objectives based on the output of their staff rather than their own output;
- there were few examples of objectives being derived from, or linked to, documented internal or external customer requirements.

Most interviewees used their own personal definitions of what constituted quality in everyday work, supplemented by (often limited) feedback from managers, peers, subordinates and end users. It was often said that feedback from one's manager was much more likely to be critical than complimentary. Acceptable, even exceptional, performance was often held to pass without comment.

An important link was made here about TQM approaches which were said to be problem-focused. Such approaches can exacerbate the way relationships between managers and subordinates could come to be based on criticism. This was because much time was spent by managers and their staff on continuously analysing problems and identifying who was responsible for them or for the processes within which they occurred. Consequently, a good deal less time was spent on celebrating the fact that other areas of work were progressing well or that significant improvements in quality had been made.

Measurement of departmental performance
Apart from technical measures of quality in departments such as pathology and pharmacy, this was an area in which the NHS sites were weak at the outset of the evaluation. However, there had been significant moves to strengthen this aspect during the period of our evaluation. The main mechanisms were the Patient's Charter, contracting, setting and monitoring standards, quality improvement groups, medical/clinical audit, and audits of patient satisfaction.

Measurement and the Patient's Charter
Some indicators were monitored more or less continuously. These included the Patient's Charter standards for waiting times; activity data including throughput; dependency measures and skills mix. Our view was that the Charter measures were still primarily quantitative in nature and geared to acute services.

The contracting process
There were three different forms of contracting. The first was contracts with purchasers, including GP fundholders. These were beginning to play a significant part in influencing the direction sites took when choosing quality criteria. Although improving, much of the monitoring was still about quantitative measures such as contact time and throughput, without equally explicit criteria for the quality of a given contact. Some concern was also expressed that there was limited or no involvement of patients or patient groups in the setting of contracts.

The second area of contracting was for non-clinical support services – for example, domestic services and catering. These services were often subject to compulsory competitive tendering and usually had the most detailed specifications and monitoring.

The third area of contracting, and one that was only beginning to be developed, were service level agreements between internal customers. There were particularly good examples of this form of contracting in the pharmacy services of one of our non-TQM comparator sites.

Standard setting and monitoring
Almost all areas of nursing in the research units had standards in place. Typically these ranged from four to 20 standards per department. In most of the units, however, nurses were becoming increasingly disenchanted with the standard-setting system and there had been little new activity over the last 12 months of the evaluation. Monitoring of existing standards was also becoming less frequent at many sites and often confined to one or two key standards.

Only two of our TQM sites had been able to set up a dynamic standard-setting process which was more in keeping with the idea of continuous improvement. At some TQM sites standards were also being set in non-nursing areas. These typically included administrative standards concerned with returning correspondence, replying to complaints and answering telephones.

Quality improvement groups
We distinguish here between standard-setting groups where, by and large, the model was still one of monitoring compliance with agreed standards, and groups which had been set up on a continuous improvement basis. The latter were encouraged to collect data on particular aspects of the performance and were beginning to make an important contribution to data on quality. A difficulty here, and one we identified at the commercial sites as well, was that quality improvement groups could get locked into a problem-oriented culture, rather than one of continuous monitoring and improvement of all processes.

Medical/clinical audit
Views about medical audit were mixed. In some areas it was said that audit groups were limited to attendance by doctors who would examine

only narrow medical issues. They were also said to be unwilling to tackle some substantive issues of variation in quality. The situation changed somewhat over the period of the evaluation. There were more examples of medical audit groups involving nurses and professions allied to medicine in audits and also audit meetings. It was possible to find examples where medical audit was much more open, including some maternity departments.

A further problem was that process improvement work undertaken by different groups was underpinned by different philosophies, methodologies and assumptions about purpose. This was succinctly put by one interviewee who said: 'Doctors rush around collecting masses of data but don't really know what to do with it and have no standards, whereas nurses get into a huddle and come up with reams of standards without having collected any data.'

Progress on departmental measures since the start of TQM

It was clear that there had been substantial moves towards, and in some cases actual progress in, implementing more systematic monitoring in a number of departments at most sites. In those areas with a tradition of measuring the technical aspects of work – for example, in pathology and pharmacy – there had been some moves to look at the requirements of internal and external customers. In the case of pharmacy, several sites had undertaken studies of what patients and their relatives wanted in terms of take-home drug services. There was also an increasing focus on streamlining processes to save time.

Some departments such as psychiatry, which traditionally had carried out little monitoring, were now making efforts to be more systematic in reviewing the quality of their work. At one of the sites this included the monitoring of statistics on each patient, the recent use of patient satisfaction forms, and monitoring of the process by which action plans were put together. A similar situation was found in some of the training departments which previously had relied only on short evaluations by participants at the end of their courses. Here there was more effort to identify what participants wanted from training, through more systematic training needs analyses. However, it did not yet include evaluating the effectiveness of training when participants returned to their places of work.

Measuring patient satisfaction

A further encouraging development was the increase in patient satisfaction survey activity, though this was, in many cases, still at the stage of discussion and planning. Although many places still limited their efforts to staff-designed quantitative questionnaires, elsewhere there were some interesting attempts to employ more interactive methods. These included the use of critical incident analysis interviews with patients and clients as well as an approach in which patients and staff in several occupational areas discussed how they thought services could be improved. The resulting ideas were turned into statements which were then paired and rated by a main sample of patients and staff, and analysed using a commercial software package.

Impediments to further developments
Although advances had been made in systematic measurement, there were several issues which had slowed progress at all the sites. The major one concerned the availability of resources for monitoring and evaluation. Resources were limited in quantitative terms often to one central TQM manager supported by, at best, one or two part-time facilitators. It is true that other resources were also theoretically available, including medical audit assistants and other staff who were on the periphery of process improvement – project nurses, liaison officers and so on. However, these staff did not come under the control of the quality department and were often operating with different assumptions about how to improve processes.

The situation might not be so bad were all staff, particularly TQM managers and facilitators, well versed in research methodology and data collection tools and techniques. At most of our sites, however, this was far from the case. Staff appointed to quality roles often found themselves there because of their strong commitment to quality improvement rather than their technical skills. Many had little or no training either in the model of TQM being installed at the site or in more general process improvement techniques. What little knowledge they possessed had been gleaned from personal reading or possibly from attending quality conferences and other short events outside their authorities.

We also noted that there was little expertise on offer from the Department of Health beyond the original technical note which was available to sites at the outset of the experiment. The Department invested considerable time and energy in cross-site dissemination seminars which provided much needed opportunities for sites to learn from one another. However, we did not see this as an adequate substitute for centrally provided technical skills on TQM or on monitoring and evaluation. It was noticeable that the support provided by the Department of Health for the implementation of the Patient's Charter was well above anything provided for TQM. The provision of a similar central service for the TQM sites would have done much to enhance their capacity to design and then monitor TQM objectives and targets.

Customer-driven quality

A major test for any TQM initiative is the extent to which organizational cultures, structures and processes have been reoriented towards definitions of quality based on customers' expectations and requirements. The idea of the customer extends to internal as well as external customers. The latter include such stakeholders as GPs, patient support groups, voluntary and statutory agencies and purchasers.

We could establish little difference between the TQM and non-TQM

NHS sites at the outset of our evaluation. Neither sample was particularly advanced on explicitly establishing and meeting internal or external customers' needs. After three years of TQM one would expect the TQM sites to have moved further on this feature. In fact this was only the case at two or three locations. The rest of the TQM sites had made some progress but so, too, had some of the non-TQM sites, the latter being driven by the Patient's Charter, the contracting process, and trust applications rather than TQM. Some of the differences between the two samples were accounted for by whether or not internal or external customers were empowered, rather than merely being the subject of an increased focus. We used this distinction to organize the following observations.

Internal customer focus
It was the intention of all sites, from the outset, to involve staff more systematically in process improvement. The extent to which this had happened depended on the amount of training, the structure for advancing quality improvement and the TQM approach chosen. Those sites that were following Crosby, or Crosby-style, implementations worked more explicitly on agreeing requirements in customer–supplier chains than the other TQM sites.

In the last 12 months of the evaluation, most sites had begun actively to investigate the use of service level agreements and, as had happened at one of the Crosby sites, this form of internal contract has begun to make an appearance. At most places where this has happened it has been driven more by the purchaser–provider contracting process than by TQM. That is, departments that were setting contracts with purchasers were finding that these could only be fulfilled if the services they received from other departments were also reliable and on time. This led, naturally, to seeking agreement from internal 'suppliers' that the wherewithal to meet external contracts would be forthcoming.

A general concern that was raised by a significant number of interviewees was the lack of a patient input to the contracting process. It was pointed out that in spite of the Department of Health's advice on involving patients and other groups (see, for example, Department of Health, 1992), few purchasers had done much to gain patients' views in a systematic fashion. Similarly, GPs, whether fundholders or not, also rarely surveyed patient opinion. It was also said that most domestic services contracts were also negotiated without the involvement of end users. Thus those service level agreements being negotiated internally were not, in the main, based on any clear understanding of external users' requirements.

Internal customer empowerment
While the idea of the internal customer was increasingly prevalent during the last year of the evaluation, many TQM sites were still not linking this to the specific idea of everybody working in customer–supplier chains. The extent to which staff felt that they had been empowered to get involved

in designing, delivering and evaluating services varied considerably across the TQM sites. At almost all the sites we were able to find significant examples of staff being more involved in this way.

At another location, a pharmacy service had backward-mapped service requirements, asking the customers what they needed, then identifying the resulting service characteristics, which finally led to standards of acceptability and a monitoring system for quality assurance. Another example was a process improvement group, made up of community midwives, who examined the process of getting blood samples from maternity to pathology labs. This involved collection and analysis of information, the design of new procedures, the setting of standards and design of a monitoring process.

External customer focus
At all sites there was a discernible increase in staff awareness of the importance of the external customer. This had been driven by many factors. However, where sites had followed an explicit model of TQM it was clear that this had definitely contributed to that shift. Where TQM had been implemented most successfully, other initiatives including the Patient's Charter and the contracting process had been reviewed in the light of customer focus and had been framed by an organization-wide total quality approach.

At the outset of this evaluation the most prevalent definitions of quality were those driven by professional and managerial definitions of service standards. This position changed markedly over the three years in all but the most entrenched of medical staff. There was now considerably more information going out to GPs, patients and clients about what they could expect from services, and this was being backed up by more systematic patient satisfaction monitoring.

Patient and client empowerment
While there was a dramatic increase in the general focus on external customers, the extent to which this had been translated into empowerment was more variable. There had been differences at some sites which appeared to go beyond individual departments to the culture of the trust itself. At one level there was a clear difference between acute units and community services. Then, at a second level, there could be differences within units where, typically, mental health services among others would be well ahead of most areas. Not surprisingly, perhaps, community services were further ahead in empowerment of patients than most other areas.

Although, overall, examples of empowerment were few in number, those we found were significant enough to suggest that important changes were on the way. For example, there were well-supported and well-organized cardiac and stroke support groups at several hospitals and a highly-regarded group for stoma care at another. Other groups which had been set up included a pelvic information support group and support groups in haematology, diabetes and rheumatology. In most of these cases it has to be said that such groups were, by and large, set up to provide information and support for patients rather than to involve them in improving service delivery.

However, the potential for a two-way involvement was appreciated at many sites and it was clear that what patients said was beginning to influence the way services were designed and delivered. We also found a range of other informal and voluntary multi-disciplinary groups. Many departments now ran pre-admission clinics, particularly in orthopaedics and paediatrics. In another example, patient care plans in several hospitals now involved comments being written by patients and, more adventurously, quality improvement groups at two hospitals were actively looking to involve patients or community representatives on quality improvement teams.

It is important to note here that although our research at the commercial sites showed that they were more advanced in a number of aspects of customer focus (see Chapter 6), the NHS sites had made more progress in customer empowerment. While the companies did consult users about some changes, there was less evidence of customers actually being involved in broader issues of design or evaluation, or of policy formation and change. There were some examples at the NHS units. We make the case for more involvement of this kind in Chapter 4 as an important dimension of accountability in public services.

One issue, which is still rather speculative at this stage but which has arisen from the analysis of patient or client empowerment, concerned the relationship between empowerment and the technicalities of TQM. This arose from our observation that the site which was furthest ahead in terms of organization-wide implementation of an explicit model of TQM seemed to have less overall patient empowerment than sites which had made much less progress on TQM. It is almost as if the increasing technical nature of the language and the procedures for implementing TQM at the advanced site have either resulted in an over-emphasis on internal processes, or otherwise reduced the opportunity for relatively 'naive' users to be involved in the design and delivery of new systems.

Quality in process improvement

It is difficult to do justice to the extraordinary range of quality initiatives that we have seen being put in place during the course of this evaluation. We will not provide more than a few examples; readers who are interested in further examples can find a wide selection in recent publications such as *The Quality Journey* (Department of Health, 1993b) and in our full final report (Joss *et al.*, 1994).

Some of the more memorable examples we came across were generated quite independently of TQM and others were to be found at the non-TQM sites. Many of these examples would have fallen short of the TQM criteria discussed above, but we would not want our critique to be seen as devaluating initiatives which clearly improved the quality of service both internally and externally. However, since we are using examples of quality improvement to evaluate movement on TQM, the examples which we looked at must, necessarily, be subject to a critical evaluation against TQM objectives.

Multi-disciplinary and multi-level effort

Although doctors have, for the most part, maintained medical audit as a separate exercise from other forms of audit (see Kogan *et al.*, 1995a; 1995b), there have been some important exceptions. Thus one medical study led to a significant reduction in pre-operative fasting on a children's unit following research which showed that there was no need to fast children for eight hours. In another study (one of several involving dieticians), a multi-disciplinary group produced a new systematic assessment procedure for the care of underweight patients which led, in turn, to better nutritional management.

Elsewhere, in geriatric medicine, a group developed a functional assessment scale for the systematic assessment of patients prior to admission and discharge, and another hospital had involved physiotherapists, secretarial staff, GPs and doctors in a study of back pain in their rheumatology unit. This was beginning to identify therapies which appeared to predict the most effective combinations of interventions and enabled the more productive targeting of therapeutic resources.

Information to users and purchasers

As we have already mentioned, all sites reported an increase in information available to purchasers and patients. However, while much of the material going to individual users provided them with more information, this still would be seen as a long way from empowering them. There could be big differences between sites. For example, at one hospital a pamphlet for the recently bereaved described what would happen in the process after a death, gave advice about how to register the death and provided a list of people and groups who could provide bereavement counselling.

However, the leaflet did not tell patients that they had a right to see the body and to spend some time alone with it, or that they had a right to see a priest or other representative of an appropriate religious group. This can be contrasted with an excellent set of initiatives on care for the dying at another site which involved the recently bereaved, different disciplines and different levels of staff putting together a coherent set of changes for improving the experience of the bereaved.

How important accurate and relevant information to patients can be is shown in the following example. A study of the return rates for patients in obstetrics and gynaecology who were the subject of either day-care or inpatient treatment showed that although there was no stated preference for either option by patients, there was an increased return rate for inpatients.

Closer examination showed that this turned out to be caused by a difference in the amount of information given to patients in the two groups. More detailed information was given to day-care patients because they were going home and would be responsible for their own post-operative care, whereas less of this kind of information was given to inpatients on discharge. By improving the information given to the latter group, the return rate was reduced.

Studies of patient need

Several studies looked specifically at patients' perceptions of need. These included: a study of the management of incontinence home supplies, and a study of the preferences of women attending a unit for the termination of pregnancies under 22 weeks, in terms of whether they preferred it to be carried out in gynaecology or maternity. In another location pharmacists and wards had collaborated with a consultant to develop a successful system to give patients more control over their own pain relief – this study was also significant for the post-implementation monitoring using a specially devised audit tool.

One of the most elaborate studies we looked at was one specifically set up to improve the multi-disciplinary handling of relatives and friends of the dying and deceased. This exemplified many of the features one would expect to find in a TQM programme – customer focus, systematic analysis and multi-disciplinary effort. Some examples of initiatives given to us would probably just not have happened a few years ago.

For example, a group of staff on an ophthalmology ward felt that too many patients admitted for operations had them cancelled because they were not otherwise fit enough. Having systematically collected data to confirm their suspicions, they negotiated with GPs and consultants for the establishment of a pre-admissions clinic to screen out unfit patients. The result was an all-round improvement in the use of scarce resources.

Systematic process improvement

A major criticism that could be levelled at some of the quality initiatives we looked at was that an important stage of systematic improvement was missing – for example, not collecting data before initiating change and/or the lack of post-implementation monitoring and evaluation. A good example was triage which in some units, through lack of proper analysis, led to more problems than it solved. However, in one unit the quality improvement group carried out a comprehensive study of the issues facing the whole department and drew on research evidence about queuing behaviour and related issues. A new waiting area was designed with a separate triage reception point, and a detailed method of monitoring incorporated.

Other comprehensive and systematic studies included monitoring patterns of demand in an accident and emergency department which produced new evidence about the predictability of demand; a cost reduction study of post-natal cots which disproved accepted wisdom that it was cheaper to repair cots than to replace them; and an excellent study of the use of medication in a long-stay hospital for the elderly which resulted in a 30% drop in the pharmacy bill through analysis of wastage and better attention to prevention.

Several examples were cited of attempts to improve the quality of catering services and to reduce costs. One study showed that the wrong supply of meals was primarily caused by illegible menu cards and an unreliable system for getting the cards to the catering department. A new system was designed with printed menus which had colour-coded tear-off strips, and this led to a reduction in the number of wrong meals supplied.

Another good study on process improvement which resulted in large resource savings was a major exercise on the provision of take-home drugs. This showed that the equivalent of two nurses' time was being spent across ten directorates in going backwards and forwards to pharmacy collecting drugs and making enquiries. A new system involving a messenger service was developed to collect prescriptions and deliver drugs. This system was expected to provide considerable savings by releasing the equivalent of two nurses' time.

Reorientation of services as a result of users' views
Although we saw the level of empowerment of users and carers as disappointing after three years of TQM, there have been more examples each year of changes in the way services are planned and delivered as a result of what patients have said in satisfaction surveys. For example, the results of a catering survey led to cooked meals replacing sandwiches in the evening; in another example from catering, menu cards had been changed after recommendations from an ethnic minority working group. In the same hospital elderly patients wanted staff to spend more time with them beyond that allowed for nursing or therapeutic intervention – now each key worker spent a full hour each day talking to and interacting with residents outside normal nursing activities.

In a community service health visitors now left their names and visiting cards after complaints that visitors did not know who they were – they also had to draft and implement an action plan about how they were going to address the concerns of clients arising from patient questionnaires. In another example from a mental health unit, staff had changed the way they tackled anxiety management as a result of feedback from patients and had implemented counselling sessions for those who were about to go out on leave.

Services for vulnerable groups featured increasingly frequently – for example, a survey of care of the elderly showed shortcomings in the management of patients' clothing and of the allocation of sexes on wards, and both these were changed to reflect users' requirements; in several places pre-admission clinics have been put on for children and their relatives before the children were admitted to wards; a new AIDS unit had been designed from start to finish by patients and had been well received.

Changes in working practices were also beginning to feature. Multi-skilling of porters had been favourably commented on at one hospital because they could now provide continuity for patients through serving meals and cleaning, as well as transporting them around the site – the porters will be qualified to NVQ level as 'service assistants'.

It has to be said that many of these projects, commendable in themselves, did not follow systematic process improvement techniques as one would have expected under TQM. In some situations, for example, visiting hours were changed because staff felt they ought to be and patients were only surveyed afterwards. Elsewhere, well-documented and well-analysed problems had led to new solutions but subsequent changes had not been monitored. However, there were some particularly good examples of 'classic' TQM-style changes. One was the establishment of a new back pain clinic which was carefully researched and staffed. The unit would be measuring the condition of patients before and after treatment in order to compare different methods of treating back pain using the TQM problem-solving model being taught and practised at the site.

Changes in health status or patient satisfaction

Few positive examples were given to us of improvements in health status. This was partly because of the difficulties of establishing outcome measures for health and partly because many initiatives had not been working long enough to produce changes in the health outcomes. However, there were one or two examples. Occupational therapists at one unit had given considerable attention to hand injuries and the development of a hand protocol. This had led to better functioning for those with hand injuries. Again, in another unit, improvements in assessment procedures in gastro-enterology had led to fewer people coming back for dietary intervention.

The evidence was clearer from the data collected in patient satisfaction surveys. There were many examples of patients reporting improved satisfaction with changes in the ways services were organized and delivered. It was difficult, in the main, to make comparisons between patients' views in the early stages of the evaluation and three years later, because of the changes in survey instruments.

Certainly when we began our evaluation most patient satisfaction survey instruments were poor. There have been considerable improvements, including the use of more qualitative techniques, such as critical incident analysis, focus groups, patient trailing, and the use of diaries and other patient-generated records. However, most patient surveys, at both the TQM and non-TQM sites, were either not repeated frequently or not carried out to track changes. Patient reluctance to complain was a continuing problem in survey work.

Part III: Summary of NHS experience

This chapter has reviewed some key findings from our three-year evaluation of TQM at a sample of NHS demonstration sites. We should emphasize that this was a purposive sample rather than a random one. However, the sites were selected in conjunction with the Department of Health in order to provide a broad cross-section of approaches and levels of sophistication at the time the study was being planned. We are aware that a number of other units elsewhere in the NHS claim to have made more progress on implementing TQM than many of our sites.

However, our sample showed a broad range of progress on a number of different approaches to TQM and we are confident it represents the range of experience in the NHS generally. Also we point out, once again, that we were evaluating TQM, not the quality of services provided by any site. A site may have made little progress on TQM but still have a high quality of service. At this stage of a TQM initiative, the reverse might also be true though we would expect that, over time, a well-conceived and well-implemented TQM programme would raise the quality of services above those provided at a non-TQM site.

The situation at the outset of TQM

Corporate approaches to quality

TQM was a pilot experiment funded partly by the Department of Health and partly by districts. It was seen as an approach which had much in common with the current health reforms, but concerns about quality of service were not such as to create the kind of climate that many commercial companies feel is necessary to drive organization-wide change – for example, evidence of rapidly falling quality, loss of market share, and increasing competition. Consequently the extent to which sites committed themselves wholeheartedly to TQM varied considerably. Only one site carried out a comprehensive series of internal and external surveys, and it is significant that this was the only location that saw itself under immediate threat of a take-over by a nearby teaching hospital. Corporate approaches (or rather the lack of them) had these features:

- There was no undue concern with quality generally.
- There was only superficial diagnosis of the picture at the outset.
- In the main, such planning for quality as did take place was separate from mainstream business planning (contracting was actually more influential in bringing these two together than TQM).
- Implementation plans, with two exceptions, contained insufficient detail on objectives and targets for any future evaluation of progress.
- Only one site set up a detailed system for monitoring the implementation.

Structural issues
The problems faced by the sites in setting up structures for implementing TQM should be seen against the enormous amount of change already being implemented in the NHS – little of it compatible with either the principles of TQM or practical issues which could be anticipated during its implementation. For example, all sites moved progressively towards clinical directorate structures which were often not supportive of TQM implementation. The main findings were:

- Other structural changes were in conflict with the structures required for TQM.
- Putting other structures in place (for example, clinical directorates or trust status) slowed down the process of setting up structures for quality improvement.
- A wide variety of quality-related groups were set up and met outside the TQM system of quality improvement groups – these included Patient's Charter groups, BS 5750 teams, standard-setting groups, medical audit groups, King's Fund hospital audit committees and divisional and specialty meetings.
- Quality managers were appointed at too low a level in many cases.
- Quality at board level was usually in the hands of the director of nursing – later seen as not the best arrangement.
- There was poor integration of medical audit and other forms of audit.

Resourcing – education and training
Although three sites had invested a considerable amount of time and effort in training, the others had carried out very little beyond some early information-giving events and/or customer awareness courses. The main points about the training were:

- Very little training had been carried out at most sites – certainly much less than one would expect to find in the commercial sector.
- Most of the focus was on awareness of the importance of quality – almost no training in the tools and techniques of TQM was provided at all but two sites. The exceptions were both following Crosby or Crosby-style programmes.
- The training invariably denied the considerable experience of research and data analysis techniques already held by many professional and technical staff.
- Multi-disciplinary courses were widely welcomed as opportunities to share experiences.
- Multi-level courses were much more difficult to manage, particularly where experienced medical and technical staff were present.
- Very few doctors attended any training – as low as 1–5% at all but one site which managed to get 30% of the consultants through the training programme.

- Courses made up of half-day events over six to eight weeks were more effective than two- or three-day workshops.
- Except at the two Crosby sites, training of quality managers was poor or non-existent.

Resourcing – general costs
- Financial provision for TQM was about a third of what is spent on typical programmes in the commercial sector. If one removes the money set aside for medical audit, some sites were spending less than a tenth of the amounts invested in commercial programmes.
- Money provided for TQM was reduced at most sites after the Department of Health and district grants ran out – at some it was now considered that TQM had been 'placed on the back burner' or stopped altogether.
- At two sites, the quality managers had been made redundant and not replaced. At a third the person had been reduced in status from board-level to middle manager. In all cases these moves were said to have had a detrimental effect on morale of those involved in TQM.

Savings through TQM
Many examples of savings made through TQM were found at all sites. These savings were often considerable, both in monetary and psychological terms. Although still in the early stages of TQM, the variety and extent of some savings suggested that an average acute unit or community service might well be able to save around 15–38% of costs found in other studies (see Joss, 1995; and Koch, 1993).

Systematic measurement – information provision
At the outset of TQM much of the information needed to make TQM work either did not exist or was not in a useful form. This is a common finding in both public and private sector organizations. The information requirement needed to be rethought. The main problems were:

- Information needed to provide evidence of the quality of processes or parts of processes was normally just not available.
- Where information was available it was often held in different information systems – some manual and some computerized. Thus it was difficult if not impossible to construct a picture of the working of systems which cut across departmental boundaries.
- The predominant form of data was quantitative. Methods for gathering and analysing qualitative data were crude – for example, in patient satisfaction surveys.

The quality of personal and departmental performance
As far as personal performance measurement was concerned, few measures were in place for assessing personal quality performance except for front-line medical and technical staff involved with very specific tasks. The main

instrument was individual performance review. However, this was seen both by interviewees and by us to be only a weak driver of personal TQM performance. The reasons were:

- Objectives under IPR generally referred to the performance of groups of staff rather than personal performance targets.
- IPRs were usually an annual event, and less than 5% of respondents felt that the process significantly affected their day-to-day behaviour.
- An appreciable number of staff had not had an IPR for as long as three or four years, while others had been in their roles for nearly a year before any objective-setting exercise took place.
- IPRs for managers set objectives based on the output of their staff output rather than on their own output.
- There were few examples of objectives being derived from, or linked to, documented internal or external customer requirements.

Looking at departmental measures, the picture was a lot brighter. The advent of the Patient's Charter, contracting, standard setting and audit had all contributed to greatly enhanced measures of service provision. Again, important developments were still required – principally concerning the development of customer-driven measures, measures which were more qualitative in nature and the thorny question of technical output indicators. There was also still a need to involve users at all levels in designing, monitoring and analysing key processes.

Customer-driven quality

TQM is concerned both with internal and external customers. We also distinguish between a general focus on staff, which we did see increase considerably over the three years of our study, and staff empowerment which was low at the outset of TQM and did not improve greatly except in one or two specific community services and a long-stay hospital for the elderly. There were a number of factors which predicted staff empowerment (and subsequent commitment):

- a separate structure for quality which, as a minimum, included quality improvement groups at directorate level;
- staff trained in process improvement tools and techniques;
- training linked to personal quality improvement projects;
- staff encouraged to review their own performance;
- process improvement contributions recognized and rewarded;
- recommendations taken seriously by management;
- pump-priming money given to teams to initiate projects;
- a proportion of savings made through TQM retained in the originating department;
- a facilitating role for middle managers developed.

Looking at external customers one can see a similar picture, although empowerment of patients and carers was somewhat stronger. Again the contributions of the Patient's Charter and other initiatives had contributed to this, though we found more evidence of patient focus, if not empowerment, at the TQM sites than at the non-TQM locations. This had been accompanied by a marked shift in perceptions about the importance of patients' views and a corresponding move towards patient-led definitions of quality. This was a feature to a greater or lesser extent at all our sites although those which had made more progress in implementing TQM had better systems in place for tapping their views and modifying services in the light of their concerns.

Conclusions

This was a long and detailed evaluation which took place against a background of rapid and turbulent change in the NHS. It was not an ideal time to pilot a major programme of change that was designed to integrate existing and new improvement initiatives within a common TQM framework. However, the fact that two sites made considerable progress suggested that TQM could successfully be implemented within the NHS. At the most advanced sites we identified five important trends, all of which showed that some of the underlying principles of TQM were beginning to find their way into quality improvement initiatives. These trends included:

- more focus on process improvement and less on environmental issues;
- more attention to sound data collection and analysis before making changes;
- a search for cost and waste reduction as well as improving patient satisfaction;
- more attention to organization-wide issues through cross-functional activity;
- a move away from strong dependence on technical and professional definitions of quality to more holistic and patient-centred definitions.

We must stress that these trends were not equally apparent at all sites nor, indeed, in all departments at any one site. Like much of the rest of TQM implementation, the extent to which these trends were apparent was directly related to the amount of training and support individuals were given for the tools and techniques of process improvement and to whether or not quality improvement structures, including groups or teams, had been set up at middle management and front-line staff levels.

Having an explicit structure for quality improvement even affected the number of quality improvement initiatives that we were able to find out about. At sites where there was no quality structure below board level, it may well have been the case that quality improvement initiatives were being pursued with the same frequency and determination as elsewhere, but the lack of a coordinating focus at department or central level meant that we were often unable to find out about what might have turned out to be important examples.

Senior management commitment to and understanding of TQM were also major issues, as was the extent to which realistic start-up funds were made available and sustained over the three years. Some sites were expected to implement TQM with little more than the enthusiasm and commitment of a single quality manager.

It was clear from our evaluation that considerable attention needed to be paid to the cultural, structural and systems differences between the NHS and commercial organizations where TQM had its origins. In both contexts, progress depended to a large extent on being able to operationalize TQM in a way that made sense to those expected to carry it out at the operational base.

Failing to acknowledge the differences between the two sectors made it inevitable that some staff in the NHS would find it difficult to accept both the principles and the implementation schedules. In particular, the evident lack of participation by the doctors was a serious blow to the credibility of TQM. In the NHS, poor pre-TQM diagnostics and planning contributed to this and were serious weaknesses. The contrast between the effort put into designing TQM initiatives in the commercial sector and what happened in the NHS experiments could not be more marked. It is to an analysis of the commercial sector's experience that we now turn.

Note

1 We have used the term *diagnostics* to refer to internal assessments of quality and *benchmarking* to refer to measuring an organization against external referents including competitors.

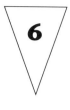

6 Learning from the commercial sector

Part I: Setting out the issues

Introduction

As we discussed in Chapter 2, the original concept of TQM and the models for its introduction were developed in the manufacturing sector from the early 1950s onwards. It is only more recently that these ideas have been applied to private sector service industries. It was not immediately appreciated that substantial changes needed to be made to reflect the differences between manufacturing and the service sector. Before applying the ideas to the public services it would be a good idea to see what we can learn from the experiences of those who have implemented TQM in private sector organizations. We can then ask ourselves, first, how relevant TQM is to public sector organizations like the NHS; and second, what modifications would have to be made to reflect the key differences between the two sectors.

In this chapter we begin by looking at some of the general issues surrounding TQM, including the claimed advantages and some of the problems which have been described in the literature. In Part II we go on to describe, in more detail, some examples of how TQM works in the private sector. Here we draw extensively on quality improvement initiatives undertaken in two companies which acted as quasi-controls in our evaluation of TQM in the NHS.

Although our judgement was that, overall, the companies' initiatives were successful, both organizations faced a number of problems along the way and an analysis of these provides considerable food for thought for those in the NHS charged with overseeing the implementation of TQM. In

Chapter 7 we return to the two questions posed above with the benefit of a fuller understanding of the commercial experience.

What can a TQM initiative do for you?

There is little doubt that a well-designed and well-implemented TQM initiative can achieve remarkable gains in a commercial environment. The evidence for substantial improvements in manufacturing processes and output is overwhelming. The service sector, too, can demonstrate striking changes in service delivery performance and gains in customer loyalty and satisfaction – witness the results at British Airways, SAS, Avis, American Express, Westinghouse, among many others. Unfortunately, few studies have looked critically at TQM in specific companies – not unnaturally, companies have been reluctant to expose the weaknesses in their TQM programmes to outsiders.

We were fortunate to be allowed to take an objective look at the implementation of quality improvement initiatives at Post Office Counters and Thames Water Utilities. We were able to interview a wide range of staff at all levels in complete confidence as well as examine a large amount of documentation. We judged progress against the criteria outlined in Chapter 4. In brief, we sought evidence of positive changes in seven areas:

- corporate approaches to quality planning;
- effective structures for managing the quality improvement process;
- wide-scale education and training programmes;
- systematic measurement of processes and outputs;
- customer-driven quality;
- commitment to continuous improvement;
- examples of process improvement based on the principles of TQM.

In Part II we look specifically at the results of our fieldwork in the two commercial case studies, but first we explore some of the difficulties all organizations can face when implementing TQM.

Problems with TQM implementations

There has been much debate in the literature about why TQM programmes fail. However, there is little reliable or detailed research about what lies behind these failures, for two main reasons. The first is that commercial companies are understandably shy about reporting problems with their quality improvement exercises. The second is that while many TQM initiatives fall by the wayside, they may well still leave a lasting legacy of improvements in some areas even if they have failed to secure an organization-wide culture of continuous improvement. It is therefore difficult to judge the level of failure. Here are some of the common causes of less than successful implementations. Although these are drawn from our research and fieldwork in the private sector they are just as relevant to the NHS.

Problems arising from inadequate senior management commitment

Although a surprising amount of progress can be made without explicit senior management commitment and understanding, it is unlikely that programmes will be successful over the longer term without visible and sustained commitment at the top. Our research also shows that senior managers (and in the case of the NHS, senior clinicians, whether or not they have a management role) must have a critical understanding of a range of models as well as commitment to any particular approach. Uncritical commitment to the philosophies of Deming and Crosby caused considerable problems at some of our NHS TQM research sites, and there is nothing to suggest that the same problem could not occur in the commercial sector.

Problems arising from inadequate attention to design

Although some authors argue that the choice of model is not important, we take the opposite view. The differences between different approaches are more profound than might be thought at first sight. In particular, the choice of model determines the language of quality, its definition and its measures – all crucial to acceptance by those working in the existing culture. Our observations about socio-technology (Chapter 3) are particularly relevant here. A further point which has been the undoing of many organizations is the lack of well-developed measures for progress on implementation of TQM itself as well as for quality improvement. It is not unusual in the private sector to find that successful TQM organizations have spent well over a year in the planning stages of their initiatives.

Managing the top-down versus bottom-up issue

Clearly the mandate for such wide-scale change must come from the top of the organization. It is also the job of senior management to give direction and purpose to the enterprise. However, it cannot afford to be so prescriptive that middle managers and employees at the base do not own the proposed changes. Cascading prescriptive training without acknowledging the existing skills, interests and needs of all staff has proved the undoing of many organizations. So, too, has imposition of structural and systems changes without consultation and involvement of those who will be affected by change. A particular problem has been the imposition of management's definition of objectives for quality improvement teams without any consideration of the perceptions of staff at lower levels in the organization. It is surprising that this continues to happen within TQM companies which talk earnestly about empowering staff.

Managing for the long haul

Although some important process improvements can be made in surprisingly little time in all organizations, and indeed it is important that this should be seen to happen, sustained improvement within and across departmental and professional boundaries takes considerable time and effort.

We have observed three stages in the first three years of several unsuccessful programmes – *evangelism, realism* and *cynicism*.

In the first stage a small group of committed staff become highly enthusiastic, probably from having read a persuasive book or having been to a successful conference on TQM. It is quite likely, however, that the support of key top people in the organization is missing and that no one has done any really deep thinking about the consequences of adopting TQM. The *evangelism* stage lasts about one to two years.

If the organization commits itself to TQM it will reach the second stage, *realism*, by the end of the second year, and this could last a further two years. People begin to realize that really significant changes take longer than expected, training takes a long time and there are some setbacks along the way. More worryingly, managers expect too much too soon – especially finance departments and boards of directors where financial time-scales are normally inappropriately short. The up-front costs of TQM are considerable and proper investment is essential. The problem is that many companies start TQM programmes when cash is tight because of falling quality, increasing uncompetitiveness and lost customers – the very time when increased investment in quality improvement is so vital.

The pressure is then to go for quick-fix solutions. Indeed, the culture in many Western companies has been to look for quick fixes of all kinds. Putting in simplistic structural and system changes in the hope of quick results is very common – witness the over-reliance on quality circles and narrow systems changes such as BS 5750 (see Chapter 3 for a critique of these answers to quality problems). Quality circles, like many other initiatives, require careful planning and implementation of appropriate changes to surrounding systems. An obvious issue is the role of middle managers who feel threatened because little or no thought has been given to their part in new quality improvement structures (see, for example, Bertram, 1993). Similarly, BS 5750 can be (and often is) little more than a mechanistic document-driven system implemented for marketing purposes.

Our belief is that all organizations go through the third stage – *cynicism*. It becomes a matter of how many people get to feel this way and how long it lasts. For TQM to be successful in the longer term the vast majority of staff must feel that it is beneficial both to themselves personally and to the company.

Education and training

Few commercial organizations start out with a full understanding of just how much education and training a successful TQM initiative requires. Many appear to think that a two-day customer awareness programme followed by tools and techniques training for a handful of facilitators is sufficient. Where wide-scale training is put in place senior managers often underestimate the consequences of the time lag – it is not unusual to find training for the whole workforce taking two years from the start of the implementation. This was also the case at our NHS TQM sites.

It is essential that mechanisms are put in place to begin some process improvement work as soon as people start to arrive back from training. The best programmes use a format of weekly training sessions where participants can work on real-time problems in between sessions. This has the dual advantages of linking theory with practice and starting to tackle some real organizational problems. Table 6.1 summarizes some of the reasons why training programmes are not successful.

Table 6.1 Some of the reasons why TQM education and training programmes fail

Training material, theoretical and practical, is not matched to the knowledge and skills of participants (leads to both under-and over-extended participants)

Training material is not linked to company's vision and mission

Training material is not linked to real problems from individuals' workplaces

Tools for improving quality are (or are seen as) separate from tools used in normal work – e.g. budget systems, communication systems, etc.

Problems identified on courses are used as training material but are never addressed by management

The difference between the need for improving cross-functional understanding (best tackled by multi-disciplinary courses) and specific problems in different functions (best tackled by uni-disciplinary courses) is not well understood or catered for

Systems to support post-course behavioural change are non-existent or not adequate

Staff focus rather than staff empowerment
There is a tendency for senior managers to talk about staff *empowerment* but actually implement staff *focus*. Thus they put new communication processes in place such as newsletters and team briefing, and give middle managers small recognition budgets. These focus attention on the importance of staff knowledge and commitment but do not actually give them greater discretion when undertaking day-to-day tasks or more power to change the way things are done in their own processes.

In some cases the opposite happens – front-line staff are empowered but at the expense of their managers. In the first example you will quickly get disillusioned staff who will give less and less support to their quality improvement groups and action teams. In the second case you will find middle managers sabotaging the process to maintain power and authority over their staff. Considerable thought needs to be given to the roles of middle managers in situations where staff have more control over their own work.

Failure adequately to resource TQM

We have already commented on the fact that TQM requires considerable resourcing with cash and training time. Many organizations start with shoestring budgets which are successfully reduced over the first three years with TQM moneys often diverted into meeting overspends on other budget items. The consequences are that quality improvement groups are not sufficiently financed, pump-priming money dries up and staff become disillusioned when they sense that TQM is coming second to everything else.

A related issue is the adverse signal that is sent to front-line staff when quality manager posts are set at too low a level, particularly any appointment made at the centre. Headquarters quality managers, for example, must have direct and easy access to the chief executive. A director of quality is preferable to giving organization-wide responsibility to a director who already has full-time responsibility for another function. Quality support managers at divisional or departmental level should be on a par with their operational colleagues. Some of the costs of resourcing TQM are discussed in more detail in our examples drawn from the commercial sector later in this chapter.

Failing to have clear structures for quality improvement

There is a considerable debate in the literature about whether to place responsibility for quality predominantly in the hands of busy and relatively uncommitted operational managers (thereby risking that it slips quickly to the bottom of over-long agendas) or in the hands of highly trained and committed specialists at the centre (thereby risking that staff will see quality as the quality department's problem). Both approaches have been found to fail in different organizations at different times.

Our observation is that at least starting off with central support and expertise is essential but that any separate quality meetings structure needs to be progressively merged with ongoing line-management meetings over a period of time. This is further discussed when we examine Post Office Counters' experience. The roles and role relationships of quality facilitators should also be clear, and operational accountability for quality in production or service delivery cannot be seen to be anything other than an operational management accountability.

The lack of thorough and honest monitoring

It is essential that, if problems begin to develop in the implementation, they are picked up as early as possible and addressed in a determined fashion. This emphasizes the importance of having thorough monitoring and evaluation in place from the outset so that issues can be identified quickly and accurately. An unwillingness to look critically at one's progress will certainly allow snags in the process to go undiscovered or untackled.

Part II: An analysis of TQM at two commercial companies

In this part of the chapter we review the experience of Post Office Counters and Thames Water with regard to key TQM requirements.

Corporate approaches to quality

Any move towards a corporate approach to quality must provide for systematic planning for quality improvement at both strategic and operational levels. One would also expect to find, over time, progress towards a common understanding of definitions of quality and the need for continuous improvement within an explicit model of TQM. Although Thames Water had no detailed strategy for quality until early 1993, this was quite well developed by the end of the evaluation. It was anticipated that it would lead to an explicit organizational definition of quality which would embrace notions of continuous improvement.

Also, although there were three different quality improvement approaches being implemented – two TQM pilots, Thames Quality Awards and BS 5750 – there were common assumptions underpinning the implementations. The company continued to work on a Deming-like model which had three stages – capturing data on processes and documenting them; getting the processes under control through systematic measurement; and then moving into continuous improvement. The emphasis throughout our evaluation was on understanding processes (the first stage).

Post Office Counters, too, had a visible commitment to corporate quality. This was well represented by having a director of quality at board level, and operations research and marketing departments which were strongly oriented towards customer-driven quality. The company also had quality support managers at middle management level at each pilot district. There was an elaborate planning process in place for TQM, accompanied by a detailed continuous monitoring system.

We were not able to interview sufficient directors in either company to form a view about how committed senior managers were to the longer-term future of TQM. However, examination of high-level documentation and the views of most interviewees suggested that there was more confidence in 1993 than in 1992 in both companies that senior managers were committed to TQM.

Forms of implementation

It is worth noting at this stage that, just as there are different models of TQM, so there are different approaches to its implementation. Some organizations set out to implement TQM on an organization-wide basis from the outset. This typically involves a major 'cascade' programme from headquarters out to all the divisions and departments in each business unit. At the other extreme, an organization may decide to pilot TQM in one or more departments in a single business unit and evaluate it before proceeding further.

Some organizations have gone for what we call the 'domino' model, where TQM is introduced unit by unit over, say, three years. A further possible approach, though not one we have seen tried out, would be to start implementing TQM in the 'earliest' stages of a company's processes (for example, purchasing in an operational process, or recruiting in the personnel function) and then extending it to later processes on an incremental basis until one had something approaching an organization-wide approach.

Post Office Counters and Thames Water adopted contrasting models. The former's TQM initiative, Customer First, followed a learn–use–lead approach derived from Xerox but adapted somewhat in the light of experiences at Royal Mail. Although piloted at first in only three districts, it was an organization-wide model which, it was intended, would be progressively rolled out to all districts.

Thames Water elected to try out three different approaches based on the perceived needs of different parts of the business rather than adopt a single TQM model. Thus the company went for (and has now secured) BS 5750 in its engineering function, an internal Thames Quality Awards programme for the majority of operational and administrative systems, and limited TQM pilots at two sewage and water treatment works. Although Thames Water was not keen to have its TQM approach linked too closely to the thinking of any one author on quality, it was clear that many elements of the design followed Deming's concepts, particularly in the form developed at Florida Power and Light Company.

Top-down versus bottom-up
Building on the theoretical discussions of this issue in Chapters 2 and 3, we can also see wide variation in implementation programmes in the commercial sector. There are two ideal-typical approaches to TQM implementation. One is the *revolutionary* and the other is the *evolutionary* model. In the *revolutionary* approach, the organization starts with a comprehensive organization-wide, top-down implementation of TQM. Participation is explicitly compulsory, time-scales are short and the whole emphasis is on achieving rapid cultural change. The *evolutionary* model is more diffuse and less rigidly controlled. The emphasis is on longer-term, bottom-up, gradual development of participation on a voluntary basis, by groups of staff who lead pockets of organizational change.

The differences are well represented in our two commercial case studies. Post Office Counters was facing rapidly increasing competition, with reductions forecast in the volume of its business. Circumstances dictated the need for a comprehensive, top-down, corporate TQM initiative with tight time-scales of a revolutionary rather than an evolutionary kind. The initial focus was on a centrally controlled, cross-functional and intra-departmental quality improvement programme, driven by centrally designed, across-the-board training and excellent information about external customer requirements.

Thames Water faced different pressures. A combination of poorly documented processes and a felt need to secure the support of a fragmented workforce led to the choice of a more evolutionary, bottom-up model. The emphasis was to be on ownership of an internal quality award programme by local line managers with voluntary staff participation. At the outset, the centre exerted only loose control over what was largely a voluntary programme of involvement in quality improvement.

However, the centre did provide general coordination and support to those who wanted it. As we shall see in a later section, both companies were forced to reappraise their starting positions in the light of later developments. Post Office Counters found it had progressively to relinquish control from the centre to the periphery, while Thames Water had to increase central control as its award projects grew in number.

Structural issues

A further major difference in implementation strategies is the structure chosen for managing quality improvement. Most organizations are agreed that, at least in the short term, TQM requires a separate meetings structure specifically to handle quality improvement. Figure 6.1 shows a typical structure. Almost all the TQM literature advises that the structure should be set up in such a way that the quality meetings structure will wither over time as operational line managers become more knowledgeable about, and committed to, TQM.

However, it is anticipated that a quality manager and some moderate facilitator support will always be required. The director of quality is shown in parentheses because only a few companies have such an appointment; more normally, the quality steering group would report through one of the other directors or else be chaired by the managing director or chief executive officer himself/herself.

It is important to note that the two arms of this structure have quite different accountabilities. The quality arm is accountable for providing technical information about quality improvement, and advice and support about implementation and quality improvement systems. It is also responsible for driving training. However, the line-management arm is accountable for identifying the issues that need to be tackled and carrying out 'corrective action' based on the recommendations of the various quality improvement groups and teams.

At Post Office Counters, the strategy assumed the need, at least in the early stages, for a separate set of meetings structures and systems for quality (Customer First meetings) that paralleled the normal line-management structure called 'Business as Usual'. It was evident that the point at which the two systems were merged required careful judgement. If the decision was delayed too long, staff complained about the additional work load

Figure 6.1 Typical separation of quality and management meetings' structures

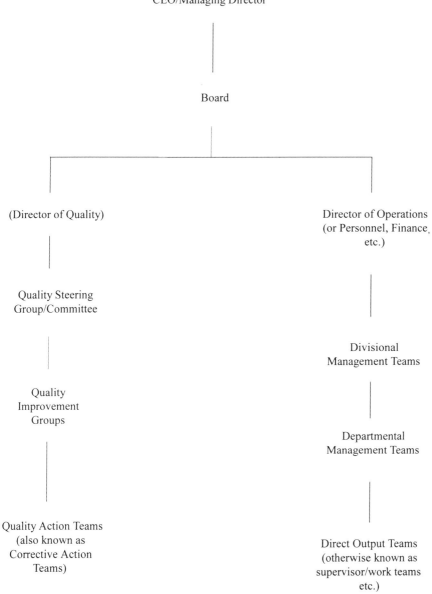

caused by Customer First. It also reinforced the perception that Customer First was somehow different from normal ongoing operational activity. If, however, the integration took place too soon, there was a danger that the emphasis given to TQM would decline markedly. There were no clear criteria at the outset as to when or how the meetings structures should be merged. This was seen, in hindsight, as something that would have been helpful.

In contrast, Thames Water had sought to keep control and coordination of quality improvement in the hands of the normal management structure, with little separation of structures and systems. The company quality manager was located within the environment directorate and reported for line-management issues to the director of the environment. However, he also had a dotted line relationship on quality issues with the chief executive. He directed a quality management team which was made up of a senior or middle manager from each of the ten headquarters-level departments. These managers held the quality brief for their own departments where they were on the respective senior management teams.

The company quality manager was supported by a quality assurance officer at headquarters and some eight full-time-equivalent quality facilitators located, in the main, within the normal line-management structure in different areas. This group of staff was almost exclusively concerned with the implementation of the Thames Quality Awards System. Further resources which could be drawn on were the quality auditors who were normally operational staff trained to carry out audits for the Thames Quality Awards. At local level, quality was handled through normal management and supervisor meetings.

Education and training

The resources made available for TQM implementation should provide for sufficient training and support to equip all staff with the commitment and skills to implement customer-driven continuous improvement. It should also encourage the development of a corporate commitment to a particular definition of quality. The training provided at the two companies during the first three years is summarized in Table 6.2.

By and large the training was well received by all levels of staff in both companies. However, appreciable numbers thought they could have done with more on specific topics. In Post Office Counters, all managers thought their training in tools and techniques was particularly good but operational managers wanted more on general presentational skills, while the quality support managers felt they needed more on facilitation.

As far as front-line staff were concerned, the general view was that the training had been sufficient to raise awareness of the need for a change in attitudes and behaviour and also to provide some basic quality improvement tools. However, most respondents felt that they had insufficient experience of using these tools in real-life situations in their own work, as

Table 6.2 Summary of training undertaken at two commercial companies in the first three years

Training for specific groups	Thames Water		Post Office Counters
Facilitators and quality support managers	48 facilitators took part in 2½ day workshop and personal development programme over 6–12 months leading to qualification as internal auditors		6-week intensive programme led by management consultants to provide one quality support manager for headquarters departments and each post office district
Managers	Introductions to own projects only		Senior managers originally had 3–5-day programme now increased to '5+5 days'; other managers had 3–5 days
Thames Quality Award staff	General awareness	1-day introduction	
	Skills training	Training not yet developed	Not applicable
Thames BS 5750 staff	General awareness	2-hour introduction	
	Skills training	Only for steering group	
TQM pilot staff	General awareness	1-day introduction	1-day introduction
	Skills training	2 days on team leadership and group-work and 3 days on statistical process control	Six modules on specific areas of TQM spread over 6 months, interspersed with learning while involved in quality improvement projects

opposed to the examples that had been used at the workshop. Spreading the training over a number of modules and months had been welcomed.

The situation at Thames was different inasmuch as staff were still principally concerned with documenting processes and had yet to get involved in substantial amounts of process improvement. The general response to training after two years of the evaluation was that it was seen as being sufficient to understand the reasons behind the Thames Quality Awards and how these were linked to the company's policies on quality. However, it was clearly not sufficient to help people with specific areas of skills – for example, writing quality manuals, flow-charting processes, or making a start on systematic process improvement. The company was concerned that staff should complete process documentation before providing training in improvement skills.

Those interviewed about BS 5750 training also saw it as a good basic introduction to the overall picture, but people were far from clear about their own roles and there was a general feeling of lack of ownership of the standard. Engineering staff views were in marked contrast to those involved in the Thames Quality Awards, who were generally positive about their schemes and felt a much greater sense of involvement.

Training at the two pilot Thames Water TQM sites had been altogether more substantial at the outset than at other business locations. However, after this initial burst, there had been little further new training (although almost all the staff at one site had been retrained because of problems with the implementation). It had previously been thought sufficient to train only the site managers and project team leaders. It subsequently became clear that it was important to provide some basic training in tools and techniques for ordinary team members in quality improvement teams. This greatly improved both commitment to the pilots and the ability of frontline staff to get more involved.

Systematic measurement

Information collection and provision can be analysed at two different levels. The first concerns the amount of data being collected through major systems. The second is at a more micro level, where individuals should be collecting small-scale data in a routine way in their own personal areas of work. These data might or might not later be fed into larger systems.

Even before the implementation of Customer First, there was a wide range of data available for planning purposes at all levels, principally through sophisticated customer relations and operations research departments at headquarters. However, the general view was that between 1992 and 1993, TQM had led to data becoming more relevant and accurate. While there was a general improvement in data about operational performance, this was thought to be primarily confined to processes within individual departments. Data about larger processes which cut across several departments were said to be less widely available. It was thought that this might improve with the impending reorganization.

At Thames Water there was almost universal agreement that the quality of information had dramatically improved as a result of the implementation of both Thames Quality Awards and BS 5750. This was because there was better understanding about the nature of processes within which people worked and there was clearer, more detailed specification of these processes in quality manuals. The main difficulty reported in respect of

Thames Quality Awards was that the production of the original manuals had been over-ambitious and it was now difficult to find the resources to keep them up to date. However, the centre was aware of this. Staff were being encouraged to prune their manuals and take out whatever had proved to be of little use during the first year.

Personal performance measures

Continuous quality improvement within a TQM framework is said to be the cumulative effort of all staff making many small improvements over time. This is thought to depend in large measure on having personal performance measures in place which encourage all staff, both managerial and non-managerial, to adopt explicit continuous improvement behaviours in their own areas of work.

Non-managerial staff

Interviews with non-managerial staff at Post Office Counters in the early stages of TQM suggested that, in general, there were few if any personal performance indicators that might affect individuals' day-to-day behaviour. The major system was annual appraisal but the extent to which this enabled performance indicators and quality standards to be set appeared to be low. Interviewees in front-line roles found it difficult, for example, to answer the question, 'How do you measure/monitor quality in your own work?' After a further year we found evidence of more direct concerns with individual performance, but development of measures was still at an early stage.

The picture at Thames Water depended on where we looked. For example, in Customer Billing it was possible to identify the performance of every individual in terms of productivity over the working day – as measured by the number of queries or arrears handled, time to process correspondence and so on. Similarly, telephonists had call targets – for example, to answer 90 calls in a day, 85% within 30 seconds.

Otherwise, the main indicators that Thames Water staff used to judge personal performance was the staff performance review (SPR) system. However, it was generally agreed that objectives and targets set within an SPR were quantitative rather than qualitative in nature, not directly related to customer requirements, and often based on departmental rather than individual performance. Some people said that they had not had an SPR for several years and most felt that SPRs, in themselves, did not drive day-to-day performance.

Managers

All Thames Water managers had an annual review but this suffered from the same drawbacks as the SPR. Although they were being increasingly held accountable for the performance of their departments, there was no detailed system for establishing their personal contributions to overall performance.

The situation for the managers at Post Office Counters was quite different. Here, there were initiatives designed to focus specifically on individual performance. The main mechanism for this was a behaviour-change programme called the Management Behaviour Feedback System. It focused on 20 key management behaviours derived from the original organizational analysis which was carried out prior to the start of TQM.

These behaviours were thought necessary to meet the needs of different customer groups, including internal and external customers. Items based on the behaviours were used in a questionnaire which was issued to the staff in the pilot Customer First districts. They completed the questionnaires on their managers anonymously. The results were then collated by the Quality Support Manager and fed back to the managers concerned. A personal action planning process followed each assessment. It was expected that managers would publish their action plans, and we saw the results of several such plans.

We observed the process being tried out in 1992, and there were some early teething problems. The purpose was not entirely clear, and some managers had either not taken the exercise seriously or had otherwise not produced detailed or specific action plans. By 1993 there had clearly been an improvement in the process. The purposes of the Management Behaviour Feedback System and personal action plans were better understood by the staff who were carrying out appraisals. They appeared to value the process and there was little doubt that it had affected the way managers behaved.

The quality of the personal action plans produced by managers was still variable but there were some good examples of behavioural change. For example, staff at one branch had expressed the view that their branch manager should be more visible to customers and should better understand their views. The manager had accepted this and set about meeting this requirement by opening the doors of the branch each morning himself rather than leaving this to the staff. He also set himself the target of speaking to a certain number of customers personally each week. Both actions had led to more customer contact.

Measurement of departmental performance

At Post Office Counters, a whole range of performance indicators and standards were identifiable at section or department levels. In branches, for instance, two key areas were identified: the first was quality of service (QOS) to branch office customers; and the second was quality of performance to agency customers (QPA) such as Girobank and the Department of Social Security.

QOS was measured primarily by the length of time customers had to wait. Individual branches were given a grading in terms of the targets set for them. Thus in one of the branches, 80% of customers had to be served in under three minutes and 96% to be served within five minutes.

QPA, on the other hand, was related to the maximum number of permissible errors set by the major agencies in respect of customer trans-actions such as the issue of road fund licence discs and Girobank matters. Branches were charged for these errors if they exceeded agency targets – a powerful behavioural prompt. Other indicators were also in use – for example, overnight cash holdings and the quality of displays and leaflets in the post offices. Sub-post offices were also monitored by staff from the area office. Data from all the branches were aggregated at area and district level. These data were published in league-table form and there were regular prizes for the best branch.

A similar situation prevailed at Thames Water. For example, in Customer Services, specific targets were set in relation to the collection of arrears, the turn-round time for dispatch of bills, and for answering correspondence and telephones. The second area was in operational performance – as in the case of water treatment works. Here a whole range of standards and targets were set – for example, the chlorine content, bacteriological content and the pH of water. It was important to note that these key measures were carried out under the supervision of laboratory staff who, although they were Thames Water employees, were subject to a different operational science line-management reporting chain. They did not have a managerial relationship with local managers.

Project management at Thames Water was one of the few areas which had well-developed measures for internal and external customer satisfaction. Typically, milestones were set for time and cost as part of the normal scheduling process, but these were linked to explicit statements of fitness for purpose. When a project was put into commission there was a three-month monitoring period to test whether it met specifications. It could also include external monitoring by, for example, the National Rivers Authority.

At both companies, there was a wider range of performance measures available for sections and departments to review their performance than there were personal measures. However, these still tended to be quantitative rather than qualitative.

Customer-driven quality

Within TQM programmes one would expect to find an increasing focus on both internal and external customers. We were, therefore, interested in the extent to which quality improvement initiatives had involved these groups at the design, delivery or evaluation stages. As discussed above, we distinguish between a more general focus on customers and actually empowering them.

Internal customer focus
It is important to note the difference between the idea of internal customers and internal customer chains. It is possible for staff to be committed to viewing other departments as being their 'customers' in some general

sense. As we have observed during our research, where this occurs one sees better communication and an increased awareness in each department of the problems other departments face. However, this is a long way from the requirement under TQM to set up formal customer–supplier relationships in so-called 'customer–supplier chains'. This entails detailed meetings between all those involved in extended processes and formally agreeing one's customers' requirements. In the strongest examples, these requirements become the subject of (normally not legally binding) contracts – often called service level agreements.

Interviewees in both companies stated that the idea of internal customers was strongly developed as a concept and, over the period of the evaluation, had led to organizational changes. For example, at Post Office Counters many departments at both headquarters and district level had been surveying their internal customers to identify both their expectations and satisfaction.

At Thames Water it seemed to us that there had also been considerable advances. Between 1992 and 1993 a fair proportion of interviewees were comfortable with the phrase 'internal customers' but were not entirely sure how it affected them in their day-to-day work. By the spring of 1993 the idea was much more widespread. Further, the idea of internal customer chains (not very prevalent in 1992) had also gained ground, and people could give rather more examples of how thinking in this way was actually changing the way they worked. Several areas were already implementing, or else were well on the way to setting up, service level agreements with their internal customers.

Internal customer empowerment
Overall, the results of our interviews suggested that the vast majority of respondents at Post Office Counters were committed to the principles of Customer First, and that their training had equipped them to participate as members of quality improvement projects (QIPs). We were less certain, however, that operational managers had the necessary skills to facilitate progress in QIPs. Also, as the organization moved towards involvement of more staff in individual ongoing quality improvement activities, rather than group-oriented QIPs, managers would probably need more training and support in managing local continuous improvement.

The main mechanism for achieving empowerment was involvement in QIPs. The opportunity to be a member of such a group was highly valued by all those who had had the opportunity. There was tension between empowering staff to tackle issues that they thought were important (thereby gaining maximum ownership) and the need to gear QIPs progressively towards business rather than personal objectives. It was becoming clear that business objectives needed more emphasis.

The move towards quality improvement activities was expected to allow more staff the opportunity for involvement in continuous quality improvement. The pressure of limited resources was also seen as a potential threat. As one manager succinctly put it, 'empowerment has no budget'. Indeed, the general attitude of some middle managers was questioned by more junior staff. They felt that some middle managers were threatened by the prospect of empowered staff.

The situation at Thames Water depended on which scheme people were in. Overall, the Thames Quality Awards arrangements had secured the greatest ownership by front-line staff, although they did not yet have the skills to move into process improvement. The better of the two TQM pilot sites came next. The BS 5750 site had generated the least personal commitment, though even here staff could see the value of the principles of BS 5750. However, they wanted more involvement in actually designing and implementing the approach. The quality manager had recognized this and was seeking ways to place the BS 5750 initiative within a broader TQM perspective.

Generally speaking, where staff had been directly involved in the preparation of manuals for Thames Quality Awards or BS 5750, or else had been involved in successful projects at TQM pilot sites, we were left with an overall impression that they had been empowered to contribute to changes in local processes, and that they were motivated to work towards continuous improvement. However they were short of actual improvement tools and techniques. It was notable that where staff had not been directly involved or where they had been on unsuccessful project teams at TQM pilot sites, there was more dissatisfaction and scepticism about the value of the whole exercise.

External customer focus

As far as external customers were concerned, there were substantial differences between the two companies. Post Office Counters was more clearly customer-oriented. Almost all its performance measures were based on customer-driven criteria derived from initial benchmarking surveys and systematically tracked on a monthly basis. Also, individual branches had carried out local surveys of around 1,000 customers per branch, and these data had led to some important local changes. The Customer Charter was thought to be an important extension to the involvement of customers.

Thames Water was at an earlier stage in its schemes and was still preoccupied with documenting existing processes. It had yet to move to a stage of relating these processes to the needs of internal or external customers, although 'work flow champions' were expected to improve this aspect. These were managers from one part of a system who were given responsibility for analysing and improving the interfaces between different parts of the processes across entire systems or sets of related systems – this is a good example of the need to tackle what we have called systemic quality.

External customer empowerment

Although many of Post Office Counters' QIPs were concerned with internal process issues, a significant number were directly related to identifying customer needs and making appropriate changes. Developments included the use of customer focus groups to tap customers' views. However, much of this activity was still *post hoc*. Customers would be invited to comment about changes already made in branches rather than being involved in the design and delivery of new systems. Of course, some changes were made in response to customers' views in a previous round of surveys, but there were few examples of instances where customers had been invited to comment on changes before they were actually made or to indicate preferences where there were alternative options.

Respondents from Post Office Counters said there was a lot of anecdotal evidence to suggest that customers were pleased with changes that had been made, but establishing the extent of changes in customer satisfaction had not yet extended to formal surveys. Those sites that intended to carry out repeat surveys had held back, pending the introduction of the Customer Charter. It was important to note that this charter was, in itself, developed on the basis of what customers said they wanted.

We observed that staff in Thames Water had some difficulty in relating to external customers because of the length of some of the process chains. It was often difficult for staff working a long way from the end user to get a feeling for what the user wanted from the service or what a member of staff's contribution should be to 'meeting or exceeding customer requirements'. While marketing and customer relations departments did survey public opinion, there was little evidence that this information found its way back to front-line staff in most departments. In the absence of concrete information, most staff relied on a general picture of what they *thought* customers wanted. This was believed to revolve around prompt service and high technical standards in water supply.

Some departments at Thames Water – for example Customer Accounts – had a much closer relationship with individual consumers, but they did not monitor consumer views in any comprehensive or systematic way. Complaints were monitored strictly and responded to promptly but there was little survey work undertaken with consumers who were not complaining.

This is not to say, however, that there were no consumer-oriented pressures brought to bear on the company. The most significant factor in the view of all staff was the Office of Water Services (OFWAT), which was seen to have influence both at a policy level and in the handling of individual complaints. OFWAT was also supported by three consumer services committees which were made up of consumers and their representatives and may be thought of as informed user groups.

However, it was pointed out that in many instances, both OFWAT and the consumer services committees were commenting retrospectively on service issues, rather than being involved in developing new initiatives or monitoring existing ones. An interesting imminent development was a move by the Director General to modify the customer guarantee scheme so that customers would be automatically recompensed for inconvenience if their billing queries were not answered within a given period of time. Recompense would no longer depend on customers knowing about the scheme and initiating claims themselves.

Progress since the outset of TQM

Both organizations had made considerable progress since the outset of their respective implementation programmes. In the main, much enthusiasm was expressed for Post Office Counters' Customer First initiative and a wide range of benefits were claimed on its behalf. Views were more equivocal at Thames Water, though supporters outnumbered those who were more sceptical. This was a reflection of the fact that Thames Water was not as far advanced as Post Office Counters in its implementation programme, and staff were not as clear about what the future held. They were noticeably more positive in 1993 than in 1992. In both companies we found, perhaps not surprisingly, that positive views were correlated with the extent to which staff had been involved in developing and implementing change. We have summarized the progress made under separate headings for inputs, processes and outputs.

Positive changes in inputs

At Thames Water, the most frequently mentioned change in inputs was the strongly expressed commitment of the Chief Executive. Indeed, staff referred to the Thames Quality Awards by the Chief Executive's name rather than by the formal title. Other changes in inputs included organizational restructuring and, in the case of Customer Services, the relocation to Swindon. The latter was said to have allowed, for example, recruitment of new staff with 'better' attitudes. The third area of changes in inputs which was seen as significant was the provision of major new systems for monitoring work in progress and providing increased customer support. These systems included a new job management system and new arrangements for account managers, project managers and help desks. The provision of trained facilitators was seen to be a major input.

At Post Office Counters, most comments were reserved for changes in processes and outputs. However, in terms of changes in inputs, comment revolved around the provision for 'management by fact'. Interviewees felt that there was a greater availability of problem-solving and planning tools, which were linked to more specific and measurable targets and indicators. This provided better guidelines for jobs, more clarity about roles and responsibilities, and better performance indicators.

Positive changes in processes

At Post Office Counters, by far the most frequently mentioned improvement under this heading was the increase in teamwork between branches and improvements in communication. Views at Thames Water, on the other hand, reflected the audit approach taken in its internal quality awards.

Gains were said to revolve around a better understanding of what the company was doing and why. Thames Water's management was generally seen as more accountable and more disciplined, particularly in relation to the management of projects. The fact that the process was generally one of social change through a bottom-up involvement of front-line staff was frequently mentioned.

In the main, employees appeared to have welcomed the opportunity to participate, and managers claimed that there was an increase in ownership of the quality of work. At the Thames Water TQM site where we undertook research the emphasis was much more on process improvement. Two aspects of the way respondents reported changes in processes stood out. The first was that they thought they were looking at all the aspects of a process, not just technical quality. The second point was that they were already looking at alternative ways of doing things, not just documenting what was already in place. This was an important distinction because many audit systems get locked into improving the documentation for existing processes rather than exploring alternatives.

Positive changes in outputs
Some of the more important gains were as follows.

Changing views on quality
Views of quality changed considerably over the two years. At the outset, roughly a third of all respondents at Post Office Counters found it very difficult to define 'quality' – the figure for Thames Water was slightly higher. Generally, concepts of quality were not at the forefront of people's minds. There was a general sense of 'providing the best possible service', but this was not seen as being definable. Several respondents in each company thought that everybody's version would be different so that it was not a useful question to ask. These vague or idiosyncratic definitions all but disappeared during the evaluation.

In our second round of interviews at Post Office Counters only two people out of 23 based their definitions on 'giv[ing] a best possible service' or 'giv[ing] a level of service I would want myself'. The rest of the definitions were far more specific and in keeping with the company's promoted definitions of quality. For example, over half the sample defined quality as 'continuously satisfying (or meeting, or exceeding) agreed customer requirements'. Five of the respondents (all middle and senior managers) also spontaneously defined quality in terms of the four Customer First principles – management by fact, continuous improvement, people-based management and customer focus.

Apart from the two small pilot TQM sites, Thames Water had not yet made any attempt to develop a company-wide definition of quality, other than to stress the need for quality in process documentation. Thus we did not expect to find as much consistency and commonality of definitions as one would find within the usual top-down, corporate-wide TQM implementations. We found many definitions of quality which included definitions based on inputs, on process and on outputs. A few staff still maintained input-based definitions which revolved around efficiency, cost reduction exercises, value for money and the proper management of financial and other resources. Here, notions of internal or external customers were markedly absent.

As one might expect, with the emphasis being placed on the Thames Quality System, the largest number of definitions could be loosely grouped under the heading of processes and procedures. The majority of respondents gave definitions which centred on defining and documenting processes. Those in engineering departments were more likely to define quality in terms of 'fitness for purpose' with an emphasis on BS 5750. There was a suggestion here that the means and the ends had become confused with, again, little in the way of a connection being drawn between requirements to improve the quality of documentation and improvements in service delivery to customers. Staff at the pilot TQM site defined quality in clear customer-focus terms.

Changes in behaviour
In many instances, changes in attitude to quality had been converted to changes in behaviour. Several interviewees at Post Office Counters were convinced that there had been positive changes in the standards of people's dress, their general appearance and their manners when talking to customers. This was seen to be the result of a considerable increase in awareness of the importance of customers, and a general sense of pride in the workplace. Three other areas of changes in outputs were also frequently mentioned. The first was an increased awareness of the importance of, and a reduction in, errors concerning agency work. The second was the evidence of considerable savings in cash flow and overnight cash holdings. The third area was in the availability of stock for branches.

Improved working practices
At Thames Water improvements in consistency and reliability of outputs were claimed to be the major benefit of the Thames Quality System. By the end of our formal research at the research sites (spring 1993) there were nearly 700 awards in different stages of completion. Some 250 had been achieved and a further 450 were in progress. This represented a considerable amount of systematic quality improvement activity. Twelve months previously, in 1992, a significant number of interviewees were concerned about the expenditure in time and money on the Thames Quality Awards and were not at all certain that expenditure could be justified in terms of improved quality. The number of interviewees holding that view fell considerably over the next 12 months.

Some of the more sceptical staff later felt that they were beginning to see the benefits in improved working practices, reductions in errors or duplication and better relationships with departments downstream in their processes. Documented and agreed procedures led to less variation in ways of working. As consistency improved, the reliability of data was seen also to have improved. Certainly, in terms of computer systems, there had been major improvements in the reduction in errors and queries from users of the systems because of better specification. At the Thames Water TQM pilot site, the process improvement approach taken was thought to have provided more opportunity for managers to understand the problems of front-line employees than was the case where they were only involved in the writing of a quality manual.

Reductions in barriers and improved working relationships
Under TQM, organizational structures should promote a reduction in barriers between different functions and groups. The view that barriers between departments were breaking down was widespread among the interviewees at Post Office Counters, although positive views were often qualified by specific criticisms. Those who were the most positive had been involved in QIPs.

Progress was seen to be driven by two forces. The first was the setting up of QIPs, particularly those which were cross-functional. Here, closer working relationships and a better understanding of each other's problems were major factors. It was important to note that barriers between levels were also seen to be reduced. Indeed, more progress was judged to have been made on this than on breaking down lateral barriers. The second driving force was some progress towards the idea of internal customer–supplier chains. Support departments, in particular, increasingly recognized that other departments were their customers. This had led to more willingness to negotiate requirements rather than one department telling another what it could have.

At Thames Water, there had been improvements in working relationships at the BS 5750 site. The biggest single change since 1992 was the requirement, under BS 5750, to have a more formal and comprehensive quality project management system. This meant that the expectations of engineers and their customers had to be made explicit and agreed formally at the outset of a project. The introduction of formal design and safety reviews allowed both sides to resolve problems which had developed. The fact that the review was chaired by an independent chairman was also seen as significant.

The picture at the Thames Quality Awards locations was not as clear. Views were mixed about whether or not the Thames Quality Awards had reduced barriers between departments. However, people were pointing to new developments which they were convinced would improve relations. The first was the service level agreements which the Customer Services Department was planning to put in place with its operational counterparts, and the second was the notion of work flow champions. These were key people working in larger processes who were to be given the responsibility for improving processes at the interface between external and internal customers and then at each stage in internal customer–supplier chains.

Views at the Thames Water TQM pilot site were also mixed. Where barriers had been reduced and relationships improved, it was because of small-scale but successful multi-disciplinary projects where people from different departments had had to work together towards a common goal. If these projects had been well conceived, well implemented and then acted on by management, then there was considerable satisfaction all round. However, we were told about QIPs which had not worked so well, and in these cases staff were quite demoralized. There were marked differences between the two TQM pilot sites (only one of which we formally undertook research at, although we informally monitored progress at the the second). One site had done quite well with its TQM implementation, but the other had more or less ground to a halt by the second year. The reasons for this are discussed later.

Problems with TQM at our research sites

We began this chapter with a review of some of the reasons why TQM programmes fail. We now look at some of the problems which even successful companies like Post Office Counters and Thames Water have had to tackle along the way.

Input issues
The issue of resourcing is important here. There was considerable concern in both companies about the extent to which more resources were needed for what was seen as additional work. At Post Office Counters, branch managers felt that they were being expected to finance training, staff meetings and QIP activity either out of existing budgets or out of inadequate enhancement. Interviewees also mentioned that cuts were being made in staff hours at the same time as they were being asked to improve quality using techniques which involved more time – for example, double-checking. At Thames Water, the major concern was the considerable time that was required to complete the documentation process properly, a process that was seen as labour-intensive.

A different issue about staff resources was also raised in both organizations. This was the problem of the cynicism of some of the older staff, including some managers. The latter were seen to be having difficulty in making the transition to customer-oriented process improvement. Managers in both companies felt that the quality improvement approaches taken were highlighting the gap between good and poor managers.

Process issues
The time things take
By far the most frequent comments concerned the delay between the programme being launched, the training taking place and 'things' actually

happening. It was clear that there was an expectation on the part of many respondents that they expected to be further ahead than they actually were at their respective stages. At Post Office Counters, another issue that raised some comment was the split between Customer First and Business as Usual. While interviewees saw that additional effort had to be devoted to Customer First, they were not clear why such an explicit split was maintained between the two areas of work. An important process issue was also raised about the use of cross-functional teams. These were thought to be a particularly good idea but it was clear that inter-professional jealousy was limiting the effectiveness of work within at least one of these teams. This point linked back to the lack of facilitation training for the people leading these teams.

Gaining real commitment

The main issue raised by respondents at Thames Water was a clear contrast between what they saw as a mechanistic and rather superficial one-off exercise (procedures audits) and attempts continuously to improve service delivery (TQM). In the former, the value was seen to lie in preparations for the audit and not the audit itself. Respondents spoke of 'learning their lines', and in the first year few felt that there was any attempt to continue improvement once awards had been made. Nor was the connection between improved documentation and improved service delivery clear. This improved in the second year as the wider context and direction for quality improvement was communicated more successfully to more staff. It is clearly an issue for all organizations whose quality strategies are founded primarily on audit-based models of quality improvement.

The fears of middle managers

In 1992, Thames Water middle managers, in particular, were dubious about the effects on their own roles of empowering their staff through the Thames Quality Awards, though less of this feeling persisted into the following year. Our research at other sites suggests that rethinking the role of middle managers is an important precursor to implementing process improvement. As staff were empowered to solve local problems and push for changes in processes, so middle managers felt threatened. They also found their roles moving from supervision and control towards supporting and facilitating staff. This was not a management style that all, or even most, middle managers were used to, and some clearly did not have the necessary skills and experience.

The dangers of a problem-oriented culture

An important issue that we observed developing at Post Office Counters deserves special mention because it appears to us to be inherent in certain approaches to TQM. This was that that the company's implementation could lead to a problem-oriented culture developing. By this we mean that a substantial proportion of the interviewees saw their model as a systematic approach to solving problems whenever they arose, rather than a requirement to improve processes continuously.

This could lead to a situation where staff coasted along waiting for problems to develop rather than looking for improvements in systems that already appeared to be meeting customer requirements. The company was alive to this issue and had begun to encourage quality improvement activities which were small projects that could be undertaken by individuals as part of their normal work, as well as the problem-oriented quality improvement groups that the company previously relied on as the mechanism for quality improvement.

Output issues

There was strong support in both organizations for their respective approaches. Thus problems were felt to revolve around methods of implementation rather than the ideas themselves or the outputs. There was strong support for the improvements that had been made in both processes and outputs.

Is TQM worth it?

Due recognition was beginning to be given to the role that TQM had played in securing better results, but people in both organizations still questioned whether the investment in TQM was worthwhile, in terms of both the absolute cost and the sophisticated and involved process improvement arrangements for what were often seen as problems that could be sorted out informally. (The fact that these problems had often existed for a considerable length of time without being solved informally, escaped many interviewees.) There was considerable support at Post Office Counters for the idea of progressively moving away from big set-piece QIPs towards smaller continuous improvement activities that could often be implemented by individuals.

The experience over the two years at two Thames Water TQM pilot sites was more variable than at the Thames Quality Awards locations. While at one site TQM continued to be implemented with some degree of vigour and enthusiasm, it had almost come to a halt at the other location. In terms of interviewees' perceptions, there were strong differences between the views of those who had been involved in successful projects and those who had not been involved at all or had been in teams or groups which had not gone so well. Some of the successful projects demonstrated to us that the basic ideas behind TQM had been well embedded in the work of the groups. That is to say, they had

- carried out a proper identification of the problem;
- collected data with a range of different techniques;
- systematically analysed the data;

- produced a range of potential solutions;
- evaluated the solutions;
- made formal recommendations for change.

Probably the only weakness in this problem-solving model was that, even on successful projects, the post-implementation evaluation was only superficially, and often not at all, carried out.

Summary of problems at one TQM pilot
The TQM pilots had provided important experience in implementation and certainly some major lessons had been learned about the kinds of conditions and systems that need to be in place before TQM can be launched successfully. These should be closely studied by any organization intending to implement TQM and we list them below:

- TQM is one of the few initiatives that cannot easily be relaunched, and therefore it is important to get it right before it starts. This means thorough pre-implementation planning and consultation.
- Line managers must be prepared to provide early pump-priming resources and then must act as role models in everything they do.
- There should be a better diagnostic phase before the initiative starts so that workers, supervisors and managers have a better understanding of the views of external customers, the business unit's internal customers.
- All staff involved in improvement projects should get training, not just the team leaders or facilitators. It is clear from the two experiments that many front-line staff had only the most basic problem-solving and statistical skills. They needed a lot more coaching and support than could be provided in a two-day workshop. It was seen as essential that each team should have a trained quality coach or facilitator.
- The projects that teams choose are crucial to future success. These should be challenging, but also manageable. The experience at Thames Water suggested that teams should not be given tasks which go beyond the site or which require considerable external expertise on a cross-functional basis, unless time and technical support can be provided. Furthermore, it should be established that there are no higher-level groups in the organization looking at the same problems. Nothing is more disheartening than to be two-thirds of the way through one's first project only to have it cancelled because the organization has decided to move in a different direction.
- One senior manager felt that TQM had been a success at one of the sites because a cascade model had been used for starting up groups. That is, the process had begun with one highly motivated and skilled group working on a project, and when that project was completed the group was split up to form the nuclei of several more groups. Clearly this would take longer than the normal implementation model, but could be useful at some sites, particularly in the early stages when there were only a few highly motivated staff.

- It is vital that teams receive recognition at early stages of projects as well as on completion. If teams come up with sensible and cost-effective solutions, they must be implemented whenever possible.
- A lot had been learned from the two pilot projects, but it was felt that one year was not long enough to understand the full learning–implementation–feedback loop.

The costs of TQM

The up-front costs of implementing a full TQM initiative are considerable and should not be underestimated. However, the question most organizations are asking themselves these days is 'Can we afford *not* to implement TQM?' The issue in a commercial setting is stark, as the spiral in Figure 6.2 shows. Given this sort of pressure, it is not surprising that large corporations invest several million pounds over the first three to five years of TQM initiatives. This is borne out by our two research companies.

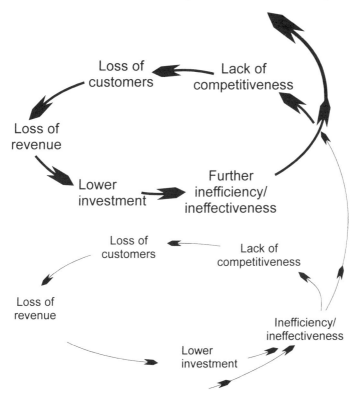

Figure 6.2 The consequences of continuing poor quality

The centralized, top-down model at Post Office Counters had allowed a better estimate of what resources had been committed. The company estimated for us that the cost for the three-year pilot of TQM in just three of its districts (covering several thousand staff) had amounted to some £3 million in the first three years. This did *not* include environmental improvements or other capital programmes. The figures did, however, cover the use of external consultants and major diagnostic surveys of customers and staff. The company expected that extending TQM to all other districts would cost a further £3 million in the roll-out year and then a further £1 million per year for the foreseeable future to maintain and reinforce the initiative.

Thames Water's costs were less easy to identify because different quality improvement schemes had been funded from different sources. There was no overall central TQM budget other than for the salaries of central TQM staff. Nevertheless, the company's figures were roughly comparable to those of Post Office Counters when calculated on a per-capita basis. Given Thames Water's increasing commitment to corporate approaches to TQM and the popularity of its Thames Quality Awards, it is doubtful that its current expenditure will diminish in the near future. The company is also committed, in the longer term, to further education and training for staff as documenting processes give way to process improvement.

Savings from implementing TQM

Given the scale of costs, one must also ask what savings will be made. Claims for possible TQM savings are often stated to be in the order 25% of revenue and 30–40% of operating costs (see, for example, Crosby (1979), Macdonald (1993), Oakland (1989)). No such claims were made in either of our comparison companies, but we were given many examples in both organizations of savings that had been made by simplifying processes, eliminating duplication, and reducing errors and waste.

At one Post Office branch, the number of motor vehicle licensing errors had been reduced from 40 in one year to one in the most recent eight-month period. At another, six-figure savings had resulted from improvements in handling overnight cash. It is important to note that while records were kept of these individual improvements, the savings made were publicized to emphasize the importance of process improvement rather than to provide aggregate figures of savings made across the pilot districts.

It was also significant that the proposed solutions for quality improvement coming from QIPs had proved in the main to have low cost implications and, in many cases, provided for substantial savings. However, managers were keen to make the point that although cost savings were an important dimension they were not the primary reason for the Customer First initiative. Improvements were designed primarily to secure improved customer satisfaction and maintain their customer base.

A similar situation existed at Thames Water. We collected many examples of small cost-saving programmes as well as one or two which were expected to make substantial gains over the longer term. Because of issues of confidentiality, it is difficult for us to report on some of the most impressive results. Here, again, it has to be said that at this stage the organization was more concerned with improving internal processes, and raising the general level of quality of both administration and technical systems, than with demonstrating a net return of savings over costs.

However, in both organizations there was considerable faith that once TQM was bedded into the structure and systems of the organization, there would be substantial savings to be made through streamlined processes and reductions in errors. This was seen to lead to expanding the customer base for Post Office Counters and, in the case of Thames Water, increasing the confidence and satisfaction of customers and shareholders – particularly important at a time of heavy investment in improving water supply and sewage treatment systems.

Conclusion – maintaining a balanced view

We have tried to give a balanced picture of the experience of two commercial companies' attempts to implement TQM. We have focused on the problems that developed, as an aid to those who might be thinking of starting TQM. We should not finish this review of the commercial experience, however, without reiterating that we were impressed with the progress made by both companies during the two years of our involvement. Those areas where we felt further initiatives needed to be made were being tackled.

Thames Water was developing a more explicit corporate plan on quality, a detailed strategy, and action plans for moving to continuous quality improvement with key target dates. It was also giving more attention to empowering consumers and securing their views at various interfaces with the organization. It was making important progress in one of the most difficult areas of TQM – cross-functional quality improvement through the establishment of work flow champions and the like.

In spite of some criticism by a small minority of interviewees at Post Office Counters, there was considerable support for Customer First in terms of both its general principles and the way it was being applied. QIPs had accomplished important goals by tackling substantial issues within and across functions. They had also enabled individuals to gain process improvement experience after their training in a supportive and coordinated atmosphere.

In the next chapter we look at some of the implications of the commercial experience for the NHS – first through a direct comparison of the two contexts and then through an analysis of some of the similarities and differences between the NHS TQM sites.

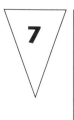

7 The implications of our findings

Introduction

We begin this chapter with a short comparison of the results from our work at TQM sites in the two sectors – public and private – before going on to examine the implications for implementing TQM in the NHS. Although the contexts are somewhat different, many of the issues faced by commercial companies are directly relevant to anyone in the NHS charged with installing quality assurance.

In the second part of the chapter we examine some of the key similarities and differences between the NHS sites in our sample and speculate on how these may have accounted for different rates of progress on TQM.

At the commercial sites

Looking first at Post Office Counters, we were impressed overall by the thoroughness with which the company had approached the implementation of TQM. The attention to pre-planning, the investment the company was prepared to make, and the commitment of a wide cross-section of staff appeared to be contributing to visible improvements in both processes and outcomes. The fact that comprehensive diagnostics had been carried out prior to implementation meant that the company could judge how well customer and client needs were being met. The methodology seemed well designed and logically coherent.

Thames Water Utilities was at a much earlier stage in its initiative and had started from a less-developed base. Rapid implementation of new technology and standards meant that more complex technical systems also had to be mastered. The company had begun by documenting procedures that had never formally been examined and which varied widely from one part of the business to another. This process had clearly been successful in reducing errors and anomalies and in getting staff to think more constructively about why they worked in the way they did. However, the company had yet to start systematically measuring and improving existing processes.

It is important to note, too, that although there were many differences between Post Office Counters and Thames Water at the outset of their initiatives, we observed progressive convergence in their implementation strategies. This is significant because it suggests that organizations which have quite different cultures, structures, systems and service outputs may still have to implement similar change programmes to install TQM successfully. The pattern of convergence is described below – for a detailed account of this phenomenon see Joss (1994a).

At the outset, Post Office Counters was significantly stronger than Thames Water in its corporate approach, speed of implementation and the results of team-based process improvement. However, as initial training came to an end and trainees moved on from their first quality improvement projects (QIPs), some of the early ownership appeared to fade. Also there was a growing realization that better links needed to be made between QIPs and key business objectives.

At Thames Water many individual quality awards were being pursued and there was considerable ownership at the base. However, it was a voluntary exercise and many business areas had not chosen to try for an award – some of those that had started were struggling, though increased training and the appointment of more facilitators had helped. One TQM pilot was going well but the other had run into appreciable difficulties. The BS 5750 site was getting under way to very tight schedules. Links between cross-functional areas were weaker than in Post Office Counters, with most effort going into smaller processes. There were few links to external customers.

Both organizations evaluated their positions and this led to some convergence. Post Office Counters began to integrate its Customer First and Business as Usual meetings structures and to reorganize using the Westinghouse model of business process improvement – flattening the hierarchy and giving support service directors operational geographic commands.

Thames Water, meanwhile, faced different issues. With the growth in the number of Thames Quality Awards it was clear that more direction and support were necessary from the centre. The company had, as yet, no detailed corporate strategy for quality although there was much visible commitment from senior managers. A high-level 'process engineering' or business mapping exercise was started centrally. The strong commitment of front-line staff to their own quality systems was seen to need harnessing to the improvement of larger processes.

Both organizations then re-evaluated their positions and this led to further convergence. By 1993 both companies had begun to implement similar sets of process improvement initiatives in an attempt to capitalize on past successes and strengthen weaker areas. Our perception was that a common set of implementation strategies and stages was becoming visible, notwithstanding the differences in starting points (the chart in Appendix V summarizes these developments). If this hypothesis were to hold good for a wider selection of companies and, most importantly, for the public sector, we believe that general lessons could be learned in the NHS. We take this point up again later in the chapter.

Comparing the commercial sector and the NHS sites

In many respects, the NHS appeared to be less successful in its implementations than the commercial companies by the end of our three-year evaluation. One should be careful, though, in drawing direct comparisons. The complex multi-professional nature of much health care work, the different cultures and knowledge bases, and the distancing of relationships between many groups, make it difficult to secure consensus on quality criteria or on organizational mechanisms for improving quality. This difference anticipates our conclusions about the need for further action in Chapter 8.

It is also clear that funding of TQM at the NHS sites, while not inconsiderable, was more than an order of magnitude lower than in the two commercial companies. With the significant exception of one NHS site, funding for TQM (as opposed to medical audit or other initiatives) was very low. Quite large multiple-site acute units were expected to implement TQM on budgets of under £60,000 per year while, in other places, units of up to 5,000 staff had only one or one and a half quality facilitators (see also Table 5.2). More worryingly, funding for TQM at some sites was already being reduced by the third year of TQM. Quality managers had been made redundant at two sites and, although the reasons were not clear, it did not look as though they were going to be replaced.

A similar situation prevailed over training. The commercial sites preceded each new phase of their implementations with a considerable amount of training. Participation at Post Office Counters was compulsory and we expected the same to be the case at Thames Water once it moved into the process improvement stage of its initiative. With the exception of two or three NHS sites, very little training had been undertaken after the first year of TQM. Most sites had failed to follow up initial awareness-raising events held in 1991. The main complaint was about a lack of training in process improvement tools and techniques. Even where appreciable training was taking place, there was a majority view that it was taking too long.

A further important difference in resources was the advantage the two companies already had in well-developed and well-organized research facilities in their marketing and operations research departments. This was one area where the Department of Health had done little to support the NHS sites. These benefits were also underpinned by a general seriousness of purpose and understanding of TQM that appeared to span a much broader base of staff than we found at most NHS TQM sites. The links between improvements in quality of service, maintaining a successful business, and security of employment were easier to draw in the commercial sector (though this was changing markedly at the NHS sites as implications of the internal market began to sink in).

TQM in the NHS had been set up as an experiment, and it was always expected that there would be variation in approaches as each site went its own way in response to local needs. However, the advent of autonomous trusts meant a proliferation of approaches even within a single district. As can be seen from Table 7.1, the general picture is one of wide variation. Only two sites had adopted an established model of TQM (both following Crosby or Crosby derivatives) although several more were pursuing Deming's philosophy without the rigour or detailed understanding of statistics that the model requires. The rest were developing their own approaches. In many ways this is to be applauded, but we feel it does require a thorough understanding of TQM in general and models of organization change in particular.

Table 7.1 does not cover all the sites (different services in an authority, and even in a trust, could be following different approaches) but it does show the differences in thinking across the sample. It also shows that a majority of the sites have changed course once and, in the case of one location, twice over the three year evaluation. Not surprisingly, the sites that had changed course were those having the most difficulty in making progress on implementation.

Although TQM is supposed to be used to frame the way all quality initiatives are coordinated and implemented, this was only happening with conviction at one site. Two others had used the more general notions of leadership for change to underpin some projects, but this did not always have a strong connection with TQM. Consequently, we found major change programmes taking place alongside TQM rather than as part of an integrated approach. Nowhere were these linked more than peripherally to TQM. They included BS 5750 where registration was being sought in services as far apart as community dentistry, catering and medical engineering. We also found Patient's Charter groups, King's Fund audit groups, medical audit groups and resource management projects in place at nearly all the sites.

Implications of the commercial experience for the NHS

For all the differences between the NHS sites in terms of philosophies, we noted that the process of change, as in the commercial examples, followed five similar stages. These were:

- a first stage where priority was given to environmental improvements;
- a second stage where professional and customer views of quality were identified and responded to;
- a third stage, which more sites had reached by the second year, of

Table 7.1 The range of approaches and changes to TQM in the NHS identified over a three-year period

Sites	Features	Origins
1	Explicit Crosby complete with all 14 steps, etc.	Crosby management consultants – 'hard' Crosby model – now self-driven by quality staff with modified language and steps
2	Crosby derivative, using much Crosby language but not explicit step leaders or his implementation stages, etc.	Led by management consultants who helped design and carry out much of the training and are still involved
3	Mostly a self-driven model of comprehensive and dynamic standard setting. Now in early stages of another change to Deming – training only but will implement in three lead departments	Management consultant led for original diagnostics and development of values, etc. Then self-driven standard setting, followed by self-driven move to Deming
4	Started with Deming theory but prescriptive approach. Faltering with loss of chief executive	Following Deming but self-developed implementation
5	Self-driven programme later moving to Deming but only in limited number of training events. No implementation in structures or processes	Self-driven 'generic' initiative but now switching to Deming
6	Strong customer service model supported by high-profile management change programme already running when TQM started	Management consultant led change programme adapted from commercial sector service model. Strong emphasis on leadership for quality
7	Several management consultants with differing ideas involved in different parts of organization. Emphasis on leadership for quality and change agents. Now considering following Berwick	Model adopted was partly self-developed and partly based on management consultant. There was a recent move to switch to Berwick but reorganization has made future uncertain
8	Based on education-led changes through empowering managers and staff in professional development groups. Detailed training packages developed on semi-commercial basis	Based on partnership with local university to develop training materials and approaches to professional development
9	(a) Approach based on training critical mass of staff in customer awareness. Sought attitude change through top-down corporate approach but little done on techniques or structure for quality	Self-developed and self-driven. Now changing to management consultant led programme after own scheme seen to have stalled.
	(b) In another hospital under same management team employed the 'Personalising the Services Initiative' – explicitly bottom-up in nature	Drew on expertise of ex-NHS consultant for advice and training then self-driven

examining processes with a view to reducing errors and waste or making better use of facilities;

- a fourth stage of a shift from process improvement to a greater concern with outputs and outcomes, particularly from a customer perspective;
- a fifth stage (still to be demonstrated in all but one site) of a move away from a preoccupation with problems in particular processes, towards continuous improvement in all, or most, processes.

Drawing on developments at both NHS and commercial sites we can make the following observations:

- The model of TQM selected and/or developed by an organization should be appropriate to the environment of that organization. Issues of culture and socio-technology are important variables (see Chapter 3).
- The order in which changes are introduced should depend on a thorough analysis of the starting point in terms of organizational structures, systems and processes; strengths and weaknesses in current quality systems; staff attitudes and skills levels; and a detailed understanding of customer requirements.
- It should be recognized that the organization will need to secure a shift towards organization-wide, customer-driven continuous improvement, irrespective of starting point. This may mean that, at some stage, it will have to implement a common set of changes.

Our conclusion from this comparison of the commercial and NHS experience can be summarized thus:

- A sense of what will be required over the medium to long term is of paramount importance.
- Senior management have to be able to provide constancy of purpose and demonstrated commitment through corporate planning and their personal leadership styles.
- Key people in the organization at all levels must have a thorough understanding of a range of models of TQM and a detailed understanding of, and commitment to, their own organization's approach.
- Plans should be supported by a critical and reflexive review process.

To this extent the commercial experience provides a valuable lesson for the NHS even though the contexts are, in many respects, quite different. We now move on to look at some of the implications of an analysis carried out on similarities and differences between NHS TQM sites.

Organizational structures and the installation of TQM

Much is made of the need to keep the responsibility for quality in the hands of line managers and this, in itself, would appear to be a sound principle. But there is little in the literature to suggest it is possible to introduce TQM successfully without starting with a separate quality structure. Most organizations we have seen, or read about, started with separate shadow quality structures, while acknowledging that these needed to be merged with normal line management once TQM was bedded in.

The evidence from this study would appear to bear this out. It is possible to say that, after three years (and in the case of some sites, four years), those of our sites which had no quality structure below a quality steering group or forum had made little progress. Where there were quality improvement teams in place, even if only in some directorates – for example, pathology or some support services – TQM had definitely taken a firmer hold.

We also found that an explicit structure for TQM enabled new initiatives to be integrated more successfully. Without this, a large number of separate groups were set up to implement, for example, the Patient's Charter, Resource Management Initiative, BS 5750, hospital or organizational audit, nursing audit and medical audit. These improvement initiatives, laudable in themselves, were based on very different assumptions and consequently were poorly integrated.

Specialty range and size of site

NHS sites differ not only in size but in the range of specialties which they offer. The broadest distinction to be made is between units offering acute services, and those offering community services. But within these categories there are great variations. Thus, one of our 'acute' sites was wholly devoted to work in cardio-thoracic problems; others offered virtually the whole range of specialties.

Although they feature in most district general hospitals, differentiation, tribalism, stratification and competition are probably found in their strongest forms in acute hospitals. Here are fostered conceptions of excellence honed within strong professional boundaries that often nevertheless allow for individual autonomy and variation within those boundaries. It was noted at several of the sites that clinical directorates based on specialties tend to reinforce uni-disciplinary perspectives and competitiveness, particularly as market forces were brought to bear on them.

It is true that among our most advanced sites in the implementation of TQM was a large acute hospital. We must not therefore over-generalize, but the difficulties for such an organization embarking on TQM are considerable. There is an emphasis on specialist quality which often demands high technical content, and views of quality will depend strongly upon their own professional and technical bases.

Size was an important factor. Smaller organizations tended to be flatter, with less differentiation. Under these conditions the range of specialties was small and commonalities between them more easy to find. This was particularly so in community services. They were predominantly led by nurses and other professions allied to medicine who could move more readily between different client groups. A closer association with communities, as a whole, combined with work which often provided longer-term relationships, were also significant factors.

Certainty and determinacy of technical content

It is possible to distinguish between those disciplines with strongly and those with weakly framed procedures. Those with strongly framed procedures might have the following characteristics: strong and determined technical content or technicity; common units of judgement; a strong frame of legal requirements; and well-defined processes (for example, pathology, pharmacy). Those with weakly defined procedures would have: indeterminate technical content; multiple and contested knowledge assumptions and procedures; and individual units of judgement (for example, administration or customer relations). We would expect the former to base their judgements on intra-professional technical definitions which would also entail a strong desire to keep control over their own criteria, whereas the latter might well appeal more to common-sense notions of consumer satisfaction, and an outward looking reference to more universal measures.

A particularly important consequence, and one which is central to our formulation of a new model of quality assurance, is that cutting across these groupings are the three dimensions of quality already referred to in previous chapters:

- *technical* quality involving technical-professional criteria in each area of work;
- *generic* quality common to all areas – for example, civility, punctuality, reliability, and respect for the worth of others;
- *systemic* quality, concerned with the efficacy of systems cutting across areas of specialization.

Within orthodox TQM, there is a tendency to apply a single approach to all three dimensions. This ignores the extent to which progress might already have been made by different disciplines and departments in developing their own approaches. For example, we noted the exceptionally high technical standards set in some clinical and medical scientific areas, complete with rigorous monitoring procedures.

However, it had been a bigger step for the more technical departments to shift to definitions of quality based on users' perceptions. There were problems with spanning the gap in technical knowledge between professionals and users. Moreover, these groups' professional training assumed the capacity to make individual judgements on individual cases. This was in contrast to the requirements under TQM to consider aggregates of cases as part of systemic analyses. Medical (and more latterly clinical) audit had gone some way towards this but was still primarily an educational tool for technical quality rather than one aimed at systematic process improvement of all three quality dimensions.

In contrast, the non-technical or professional disciplines at the other end of the spectrum had been more amenable to improving generic and sys-temic issues but had little or no tradition of rigorous measurement. They needed more help with this aspect than was provided within what was, by and large, inadequate training and technical support on measurement techniques. It was noticeable, too, that those responsible for implemen-ting quality improvement, including planning and quality departments, did little monitoring of their own work.

The analysis demonstrates that considerably more thought needs to be given to how different disciplines and departments might be more effec-tively convinced of the need for improvements in all three dimensions of quality and, once convinced, supported in developing the requisite quality assurance systems. An alternative model for quality assurance is presented in Chapter 8.

Change and implementation models

As we have noted in Chapter 3, several patterns are proposed for caus-ing change. Here we focus on two of the most important – bottom-up and top-down approaches, and forward mapping as opposed to backward mapping.

Top-down versus bottom-up

The most often used phrase in our sites was that quality systems are top-led and bottom-fed. In practice, however, for the most part the reiterative interaction between levels that this phrase implies did not exist. All sites were to some extent working on a top-down model, but, as we have seen in Chapter 5, the extent of senior management commitment and active leadership was mostly unimpressive. The majority of initiatives were started at the base. They were not then well connected with other levels of the organization, and did not form part of a total organizational quality ini-tiative through specification of objectives and techniques or by the alloca-tion of resources. Most of the sites employed quality facilitators or managers, but their role was that of educator and facilitator without staff authority fully to inaugurate and monitor action.

Our analysis of the differences between top-down and bottom-up ar-rangements is summarized in Table 7.2. The data are drawn primarily from one provider unit that was implementing each approach in different units on a split site. However, the results are supported by more general findings in the TQM literature.

Forward mapping and backward mapping

It follows from the above description of top-down initiatives that there was little or no mapping of either kind as far as quality objectives were concerned. The general organizational model, however, was one of forward

Table. 7.2 A comparison of bottom-up and top-down approaches

Common Axes	Bottom-up	Top-down
Breadth versus depth	Tend to be uni-disciplinary, inward looking, isolated teams. Narrow breadth but greater vertical penetration	Tend to be more corporate, more multi-disciplinary, outward-looking and more likely to be integrated with organizational objectives. Much less penetration after three years, except where full directorate quality structures have been put in place
Approaches and activities	Mainly reactive, problem-focused, concerned with generic issues, entrepreneurial and based on personal interests. Mainly focused on improving environment though this changed somewhat in year 3	More proactive and systemic. More likely to be looking at cross-functional issues. Strong managerial content
Commitment and awareness	Senior management – high	Senior management – high
	Middle management – low	Middle management – moderate
	Junior staff – high	Junior staff – low
Issues	Potential for inward-looking teams	Long implementation
	Preponderance of very enthusiastic staff but under-skilled in quality techniques	Organizational drag and cynicism could build up
	Lack of coordination and some duplication/ inconsistency	High levels of rumour in absence of detailed progress reports
	Concern by middle managers that they were losing control	Lack of consultation with junior staff by management
	Failure by some managers to recognize and reward individual efforts	Lack of ownership of aims/ objectives by staff at base
	Staff felt that at least the changes were actually required	

mapping of organizational change. Objectives were set at the top but in most sites implementation was not achieved through the phased application of specific techniques. Most of the initiatives were started outside the TQM pilots at the point where practitioners worked with their clients. For the most part these were not brought together into a total organization scheme or worked through layers of organization and ultimately adopted by the top. Some forward mapping was evident in a minority of cases where it was felt that a culture shift had been secured through the pursuit of specific problems and the monitoring of their solution.

There was little evidence of backward mapping when it came to identifying the needs of patients and other users before initiating organizational change. While more information was going out to patients, and more attention being paid to securing views about existing systems and processes, less effort was being expended on consulting about proposed changes or in involving users in designing and developing new services.

Empowerment of staff and users

This factor depended more on the modes of implementation than on the concepts behind some of the approaches. For example, Deming's model was applied in quite different ways at three sites. At one it was being used as a training mechanism for increasing understanding of the need to measure variation, with little implementation in practice. At a second, it was also being used in training but plans were in hand progressively to install it in three lead directorates once it had been developed and negotiated with key medical staff. At the third location, it was being implemented in a highly prescriptive and top-down way. Empowerment of users was not a significant feature of the way Deming was being implemented at any of these sites although other (unconnected) quality improvement activity did empower users in some departments.

The Crosby approach involved a considerable number of staff in interesting and highly effective quality projects at a small community hospital but was significantly less effective at the larger acute unit. It required well-developed relationships and a prior willingness to tackle some substantial and long-standing areas of error and waste. It was led by a charismatic consultant and this certainly helped the process.

The implementation of a Crosby-type approach at a second large acute unit was the most successful of all, which shows that this approach can work given the right circumstances. A considerable number of staff were involved in improvement activity. The differences between this location and others included the annual expenditure on external consultancy support and training (well into six figures), the commitment of the Chief Executive, and an effective and persevering quality manager who had come from the pharmaceutical sector.

However, it is significant that the empowerment of users was lower here than at nearly all our other sites. We speculate that this may be an unfortunate side-effect of having a well-developed and technically strong TQM programme – it reduces the chance of 'naive' users getting involved because they are not familiar with the detailed technical aspects of process improvement.

The other approaches, including the softer leadership and self-developed approaches, appeared, on the face of it, to provide for greater empowerment of staff. However, in many cases, it reached only a limited number of people. It was apparent that the approach needed more structure and direction in order to get more people involved.

Empowerment of patients and carers was weak at most sites although we found some significant exceptions everywhere. These examples, however, were often the result of dedicated effort by individuals or small groups with a particular interest in a single client group. TQM did little to promote empowerment of users.

Summary and conclusions

From all that we have already said, it will be clear that:

- all organizations, private and public (including the NHS) have quality concerns which give rise to common problems;
- at the same time, the nature of the tasks to be performed gives rise to different values, styles of work and organizational patterns;
- it is essential that arrangements for quality assurance reflect these differences and avoid importing what will be seen as an alien culture and system.

In the first part of the final chapter we show how 'orthodox' TQM could be refined to take account of the issues we have identified in preceding chapters. However, we feel that even an improved orthodox model still falls short of what could be achieved by installing a more radical mixed model of quality assurance. We conclude the final chapter with a description of the new model and the implications for its installation.

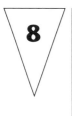

8 Agenda for reform

In this book we have been concerned primarily to help practitioners and managers come to grips with concepts of quality and ways of applying them to their own zone of work within the NHS.

We know from our evaluation of the pilot schemes in the NHS that while health service employees have much to learn from the considerable body of thought about quality to be found in the TQM literature, it needs to be applied carefully and selectively. Before putting time and effort into creating a system of quality assurance, it is essential to be clear which of the many concepts of quality one is adopting (see Chapter 2). Then the practical problems involved in applying the chosen approach to a particular zone of work have to be faced. Thought must also be given to ensuring that it is applied comprehensively throughout what are, in the NHS, complex organizations.

In this chapter we begin by describing how it is possible to improve on efforts to implement 'orthodox' TQM in the NHS, of the kind described in Chapter 2. We then go on to offer our own Brunel quality model (BQM).

Following the gurus: installing orthodox TQM

There are many conflicting definitions of TQM. You will recall that our composite definition of orthodox TQM is *an integrated, corporately-led programme of organizational change designed to engender and sustain a culture of continuous improvement based on customer-oriented definitions of quality.*

Given this definition, what factors might lead to significant movement towards this form of TQM? In our fieldwork we analysed them at two points in time. Table 8.1 shows the main factors that we found consistently predicted progress.

Table 8.1 Factors which predict significant TQM movement

Demonstrated senior management commitment to, and understanding of, TQM

A well-developed and well-documented implementation strategy put in place, with clear objectives, time-scales, action plans, and review mechanisms

Strong/persevering TQM coordinator with excellent communication skills; board-level appointment or at least direct access to chief executive

Sufficient funding for adequate number of TQM facilitators. Experience suggests a requirement for about one per 500 staff at business manager/service manager level

A full shadow structure for overseeing implementation of TQM. Strategy for integrating this with normal line-management meetings as soon as managers are trained and continuous improvements has moved out from quality improvement teams to majority of front-line staff

Comprehensive pre-TQM review of service quality plus views of staff, users, purchasers, competitors. Then continuous monitoring of key customer criteria

Early effort to gain support of medical consultants using survey data. Stronger links between different forms of audit

Standard setting but only part of strongly monitored continuous improvement

Comprehensive TQM training using mixed classroom/workplace practice model. To be attended by staff at all levels including medics and the board. Training to cover tools and techniques, not just awareness

Explicit strategy/resources for recognizing/rewarding progress on TQM

Changes to organizational structures and systems only made after careful evaluation using principles of TQM. Must include consultation with staff, end users and other stakeholders

---

Source: based on Joss *et al.* (1992, p. 54).

It is difficult to say which of these factors are the most important. Our observation of quality assurance at Post Office Counters and Thames Water certainly suggests that the order in which factors emerge is important. For example, the support and skills of senior management are crucial early on, whereas training in technical skills becomes increasingly important if initiatives are not to stall at a later stage.

So, in offering a discussion of each factor we emphasize the importance of each in its own right but cannot make any reference to any multiplier effect that might be possible.

Demonstrated senior management commitment by all senior managers

We share the view of other writers on TQM that this factor is of central importance but stress the word 'demonstrated'. During our research, interviewees repeatedly commented on the difference between the rhetoric of quality and what they saw as a lack of demonstrated commitment. They contrasted statements made in trust applications and bids for Department of Health moneys with the reality of day-to-day performance by senior managers. The most frequent examples of what was meant by demonstrated commitment included:

- spending time 'walking the job' for explicit quality improvement purposes and insisting on what we have called generic quality – being on time for meetings and keeping promises;
- setting quality improvement objectives for their own performance and publishing the results;
- opening and closing training courses on quality improvement (which should be attended by senior managers and clinicians) and being prepared to answer difficult questions about quality and lack of resources;
- showing a strong presence at quality presentations and open days;
- chairing top quality committees rather than delegating responsibility;
- being prepared to undergo training in TQM tools and techniques.

Full understanding of TQM by senior managers and clinicians

It was clear from our research that demonstrated commitment without full understanding of TQM was insufficient to produce top-led change. We found, for example, some committed senior staff at one Crosby site who, two years after the start of their initiative, did not realize that there were alternative approaches to TQM. They had little knowledge of the fairly serious critiques that had been mounted against Crosby's approach. Their main concern was with acceptability of Crosby's language, not his philosophy. In another case, we observed that an over-zealous commitment to a single approach (this time Deming), and a determination to install it at all costs, had had a damaging effect on people's willingness to involve themselves in TQM.

Managers, from the chief executive downwards, should have a broad understanding of different models of TQM and a detailed understanding of the advantages and disadvantages of the model proposed for their own organization. It should be possible for them to pursue quality improvements in a determined way (particularly relating to generic and systemic quality) while still maintaining intellectual speculative doubt about TQM as a concept.

Pre-planning and a documented corporate planning system

TQM implementations require careful and detailed pre-planning. They are intended to make coherent and integrated alterations to the culture, structure and systems of an organization. The planning stage at all except two demonstration sites in the TQM experiments was relatively short and superficial. In part this was because they needed to meet Department of Health time-scales; the main deficit was in detailed understanding of the concepts and implementation requirements of TQM.

Monitoring and evaluation of the implementation are needed from the outset. A significant difference between Post Office Counters and the NHS sites was the time they spent in pre-planning on TQM. This enabled Post Office Counters to have a clear idea about where it wanted to go and what needed to be done to get there. The company was also more able to integrate the many different organizational initiatives already in the pipeline.

A further important difference was the effort Post Office Counters put into developing and then installing systems for evaluating progress on its TQM implementation (in addition to measures of the quality of services). There was a greater preparedness to accept and tackle shortcomings in its implementation plans.

Pre-TQM diagnostics and benchmarking

If the implementation of TQM is to be consistent with its own principles, it should be based on an accurate understanding of the organization's needs. To take one of the most important objectives as an example, the TQM principle of customer-driven quality implies that initiatives should be based on genuine consultations with staff, end users and other stakeholders. Comprehensive pre-TQM diagnostics and benchmarking should then lead to well-developed and well-documented implementation strategies with clear statements of aims, goals, objectives, targets and plans.

A number of diagnostic tools are used in the TQM world for assessing progress on quality improvement and, with modification, these would serve as a useful starting point for the NHS. One of the earliest, *the quality management maturity grid*, was provided by Crosby (1979, pp. 32–3). This provided six five-point scales on issues to do with management attitude, organizing for quality, and problem handling.

A more recent and fuller set of criteria come from the Malcum Baldridge National Quality Award. This prestigious award was established in the United States in 1987 with a view to promoting the quality achievements of U.S. companies. Since then the criteria on which the award is based have formed the basis of many other audit systems around the world. Several of the award's criteria are used by Post Office Counters and, although they are not specific to public sector health care, a relevant set could easily be devised. We have developed a chart (Appendix VI) which can be used diagnostically to review the current state of quality systems in a typical health unit. This links to our models for vertical and lateral audit discussed below.

Structuring for quality

Almost all the research sites felt that it was essential to have a total quality manager or coordinator in a central role. This person would need excellent communication skills, charisma and perseverance. He or she should have easy and direct access to the chief executive and should report to someone at board level who has a specific quality brief. Although, traditionally, quality at board level has been part of the brief of the director of nursing, there is now increasing support for the view that quality would be more appropriately combined with a broader director of contracting role.

Opinions were divided about the most appropriate structure for handling quality improvement issues in directorates. There was a tension between having a separate quality structure (thereby potentially creating the notion that quality was mainly the business of the quality department), and leaving responsibility for quality improvement in the hands of line managers (with the potential for its slipping ever further down busy managers' agendas).

The majority view at our NHS and commercial sites was that accountability for continuous quality improvement should remain with line managers and other staff but that, in the early stages of TQM, staff should be supported by technical expertise provided by a centrally coordinated quality team. This would include roles at junior or middle management level for TQM facilitators located in directorates.

NHS sites that have followed this model have made more progress in getting the ideas of TQM from senior management down to front-line staff. They have also been more successful in ensuring that quality improvement projects are coordinated and in keeping with the particular TQM approach chosen by the organization. We have seen little to suggest that understanding or implementation of TQM has taken root where sites have given line managers the main responsibility for quality improvement without the support of any shadow structure at directorate level. Middle managers do need the support of a full- or part-time quality facilitator in the first two to three years.

Our best estimate, after observing three years of TQM, is that a new TQM site should be thinking in terms of a ratio of about one facilitator to 500 staff. These facilitators need not be full-time but should be available on a genuine part-time basis (not the usual arrangement where they are expected to manage TQM in addition to a full-time job). Larger directorates should, therefore, have their own facilitator, while smaller ones could share.

Where an organization started with separate management meetings for quality and main-line business, there seemed to be general agreement that these meetings should progressively merge until discussions about quality issues become a standing part of normal line-management meetings. However, it was likely that there would still be a need for support from directorate quality teams and a central TQM coordinator.

The role to be played by quality staff in directorates was far from clear and caused difficulties at several sites. Many middle managers already felt under threat from the requirement to empower their staff and were not keen to have another person at supervisor or management level who would facilitate quality improvement projects in their own departments.

In all our sites, directorate-level quality staff met with the central quality manager who, in turn, had access to the chief executive. This provided a route from front-line staff to the board on quality (and non-conformance) issues which by-passed the management chain. It is important to reach agreement on whether quality staff are in predominantly staff roles acting on behalf of the clinical director, whether they are outposted from the central quality department, and whether they have a strong monitoring role or not.

Our view is that they should be in the directorate structure and managed by service directors, but also have a reporting relationship with the central quality manager on technical issues of quality. They would coordinate and monitor rather than have a direct management function. Their main role would be to

- encourage new quality improvement activity;
- coordinate it with other initiatives;
- assist directorate staff to develop monitoring and evaluation systems for quality assurance.

Involving staff, including the doctors

One can hardly claim to be implementing TQM as long as a large and influential group of staff remain uninvolved. Given the way junior doctors are trained, which is unlikely to change substantially in the near future, it is essential that permanent and senior medical staff are committed to the basic principles of TQM.

It was clear from our study that this depended on securing the cooperation of key clinicians at an early stage, certainly before schemes had been launched. The longer this was left, the more difficult it subsequently proved to be. Some of the later antagonism was not surprising since implementation of TQM meant quite junior non-medical staff collecting data on doctors' performance as part of systematic process improvement activity. Moreover, highly trained professionals, used to administering their own quality criteria, will need convincing of the need for generic and systemic forms of quality assurance.

The chief executive at one of the few sites in our sample that had managed to secure cooperation of significant numbers of doctors put his success down to his long-standing and cordial relationships with the medical director and the chair of medical audit. It seems likely that it would be difficult to initiate TQM without the active support of these two figures.

Two important factors appeared to contribute to getting senior clinicians involved. The first was involvement in the pre-planning phase, including workshop-style strategic planning and training events. The second was the use of survey data from diagnostics and benchmarking results to make clinicians more aware of the expectations and requirements of key internal and external customers.

The change in the general climate since the beginning of our evaluation should now make it easier to involve doctors in TQM. The process of securing trust status, of convincing purchasers and GP fundholders that the organization can meet quality standards, and the advent of the Patient's Charter have all contributed to raising the awareness of the importance of structured and continuous quality improvement.

In spite of this new climate, it was still the case that the majority of consultants had little if any involvement in TQM at the research sites. While one of our sites did achieve a 30% attendance of consultants at TQM training events, the other sites had an attendance of only 1–5%. It was also almost impossible to secure their attendance at quality improvement team meetings. Although time pressures were obviously a factor, it was clear that most doctors were unprepared to make much effort to get involved. This was either because they disagreed with the principles of TQM or with the way it was being implemented locally (or both).

The change model implied by TQM requires persuasion by evidence and the logic of quality assurance. Our impression was that gathering and disseminating information about process variation in service delivery increasingly intrigued doctors who were part of those processes. Involving them in collecting, analysing and interpreting the data was an important precursor to getting them to change working practices. This tactic was one of the reasons why the Deming approach to TQM was relatively well received by doctors at sites that were restarting their initiatives with this approach.

Continuous quality improvement

Continuous quality improvement through attention to processes lies at the heart of all models of TQM. There are two aspects to this. The first is deciding whose definitions of quality the organization will follow. In the commercial sector this is quite clear – the customer is said to be the ultimate arbiter of quality and the organization's structure, systems, processes and people require realignment to 'delight customers by continuously meeting and where possible exceeding agreed requirements'.

The situation in the public sector in general, and in health in particular, is more complex. There are numerous stakeholders involved in service delivery and they may have different views about quality – some will not even be receiving the services voluntarily. As Øvretveit (1992) has pointed out, there are at least three important dimensions to quality of health services – professional quality, client quality and management quality. The definition of customers would have to include users, purchasers and a whole range of pressure groups and agencies.

If one adds our elements of quality – generic, systemic and technical (these have something in common with Øvretveit's classification but refer more to components of quality assurance) – it can be seen that reaching an accommodation between stakeholders will be difficult indeed.

The second factor concerns the arrangements for process improvement activity itself. TQM requires a dynamic model of monitored continuous improvement in all work processes. This was markedly absent at most of our research sites. The standard-setting process, even that proposed in the RCN's Dynamic Standard Setting System, was not, by and large, compatible with the principles of continuous improvement. Standards had generally been set as minimally acceptable markers of good practice which were then audited, at best, once or twice a year. Providing they were met, many would remain in place unchanged for several years. Only one of our sites systematically tightened criteria if they were met in successive quarterly audits.

The fact that doctors continued to see medical audit as an activity quite separate from, but complementary to, other forms of audit had not helped. However, it may well be that the NHS Management Executive's intention to shift funding from doctor-led medical audit to management-led clinical (process) audit will encourage a shift towards integrated audit of complete processes.

Lateral audit
In Figure 8.1 one can see how a typical example of an excellent medical audit study had repercussions that went well beyond the doctors. A small but significant change in medical practice in outpatients caused considerable problems for nursing practice, the sterile supplies, pharmacy services and management, because thought had not been given to the implication of the change on other systems.

This example indicates the need for a mechanism to bring together key people from each of the main audit areas to follow through on proposed changes. The format for this will differ at each site depending on how the quality structure has been set up. It may be facilitated when the shift from medical to clinical audit is complete.

Vertical audit
Figure 8.2 describes one set of links for improving on vertical integration of different audits. It takes into account some of the main weaknesses we observed in audit arrangements at some of the sites. First, and most importantly, it describes what some of the key differences should be between the quality improvement activities at each level. Starting at the base, individuals and small teams are mainly concerned with improving performance

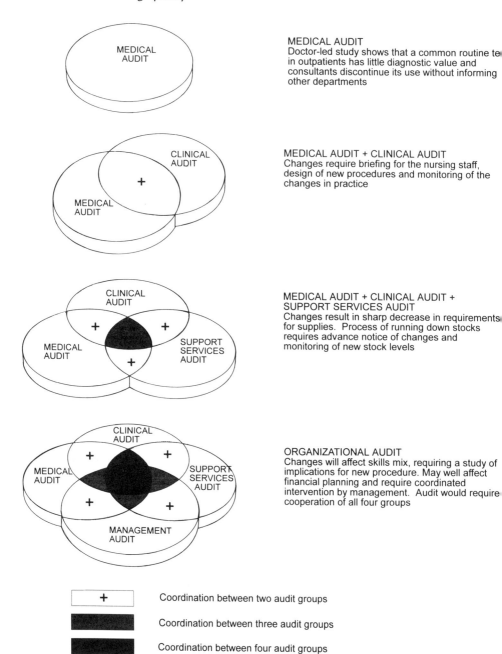

MEDICAL AUDIT
Doctor-led study shows that a common routine te
in outpatients has little diagnostic value and
consultants discontinue its use without informing
other departments

MEDICAL AUDIT + CLINICAL AUDIT
Changes require briefing for the nursing staff,
design of new procedures and monitoring of the
changes in practice

MEDICAL AUDIT + CLINICAL AUDIT +
SUPPORT SERVICES AUDIT
Changes result in sharp decrease in requirements
for supplies. Process of running down stocks
requires advance notice of changes and
monitoring of new stock levels

ORGANIZATIONAL AUDIT
Changes will affect skills mix, requiring a study of
implications for new procedure. May well affect
financial planning and require coordinated
intervention by management. Audit would require
cooperation of all four groups

Coordination between two audit groups

Coordination between three audit groups

Coordination between four audit groups

Figure 8.1 An example of lateral arrangements needed to manage a change
affecting several departments

in discrete episodes and tasks. At the next level there is a shift to managing flows of work and analysing aggregate sets of data about processes with a view to improving them. Activity is mainly within individual departments.

The next level, and one which is still particularly weak, is the activity concerned with improving cross-functional processes. The complex specialty structure, reinforced now by clinical directorates, has improved arrangements for quality improvement within departments, but we were told in some places that this had been to the detriment of better working between departments. The trust-wide quality forum in the third tier in Figure 8.2 should be expressly concerned with this issue, rather than dealing with individual quality projects as has often been the case in the past.

The final level is the board, where we see the key input as the development and promotion of an organization-wide culture of continuous improvement. This requires a reorientation of all the structures and systems to provide the right environment within which continuous quality improvement can thrive. It is essential that the board demonstrates its commitment to CQI through improving the quality of its own work as well as through communicating the importance of quality to lower levels.

The second feature of the model is the lateral integration of quality improvement groups at each level as described above. Again, it is important to note that the groups coming together at each level must be made up of those with authority and accountability for action at the respective levels. There is little point in a clinical director, who has accountability for cross-directorate process improvement, delegating responsibility for this to a staff member in the next level down when that person will not have the authority to make substantive changes.

The third suggestion is based on the notion of 'nested team management'. This is a method whereby one person from the groups at each level sits on the group in the level above. This speeds up communication between the levels. How this is organized will depend on the size and number of groups at each level.

Taking account of clinical audit arrangements

In a comprehensive study of clinical audit, Kogan *et al.* (1995a; 1995b) have described the complex inter-related cycles that need to be taken into account when searching for better integration of audits. They considered the relationships between the patient care cycle, the standard-setting cycle, and the clinical audit cycle. They also built into their analysis a cycle concerned with securing agreement to systems changes.

Although the authors were looking specifically at four health professions, we see their analysis as being relevant to a more general debate about audit systems. We have reinterpreted some of their work in order to arrange their cycles within the model of different organizational levels used earlier. This further analysis produces the results shown in Figure 8.3. The numbering of stages in each cycle corresponds to those in Kogan *et al.* (1995a, Figure 11.1).

Figure 8.2 A model for vertical integration of quality audits

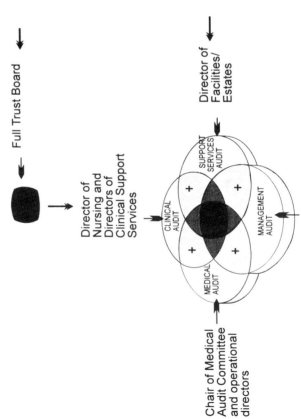

Strategic level
Trust Board integrates directorate-level business and quality plans into corporate plan. Time-scale: 5–10 years ahead

(One person from each group sits on next level up)

Cross-functional integration
Organization-wide quality forum facilitates quality planning process across directorates. Focus is on cross-functional process improvement. Time-scale: 2–5 years ahead

Full Trust Board

Director of Nursing and Directors of Clinical Support Services

Director of Facilities/ Estates

Chair of Medical Audit Committee and operational directors

CLINICAL AUDIT

SUPPORT SERVICES AUDIT

MEDICAL AUDIT

MANAGEMENT AUDIT

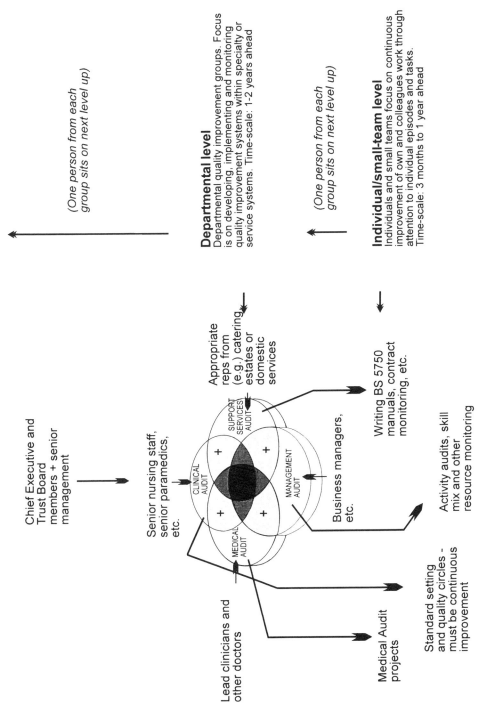

Departmental level
Departmental quality improvement groups. Focus is on developing, implementing and monitoring quality improvement systems within specialty or service systems. Time-scale: 1-2 years ahead

(One person from each group sits on next level up)

Individual/small-team level
Individuals and small teams focus on continuous improvement of own and colleagues work through attention to individual episodes and tasks.
Time-scale: 3 months to 1 year ahead

(One person from each group sits on next level up)

Chief Executive and Trust Board members + senior management

Senior nursing staff, senior paramedics, etc.

Appropriate reps from (e.g.) catering estates or domestic services

Writing BS 5750 manuals, contract monitoring, etc.

Business managers, etc.

Activity audits, skill mix and other resource monitoring

Lead clinicians and other doctors

SUPPORT SERVICES AUDIT

CLINICAL AUDIT

MANAGEMENT AUDIT

MEDICAL AUDIT

Medical Audit projects

Standard setting and quality circles - must be continuous improvement

Figure 8.3 A reworked version of Kogan *et al.*'s (1995a) analysis of different cycles in the clinical audit process

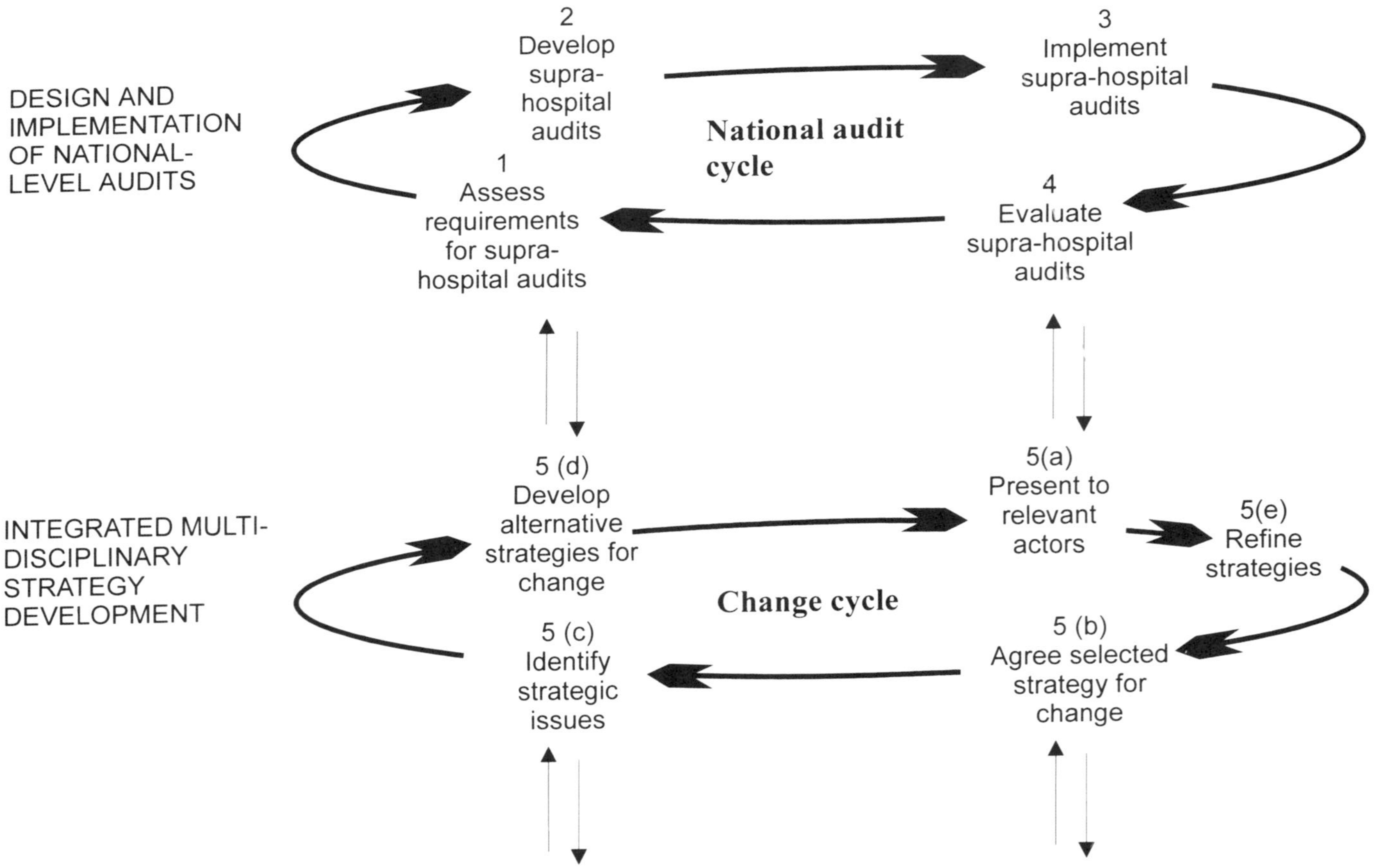

National audit cycle

2
Develop supra-hospital audits

3
Implement supra-hospital audits

4
Evaluate supra-hospital audits

1
Assess requirements for supra-hospital audits

DESIGN AND IMPLEMENTATION OF NATIONAL-LEVEL AUDITS

Change cycle

5(a)
Present to relevant actors

5(e)
Refine strategies

5 (b)
Agree selected strategy for change

5 (c)
Identify strategic issues

5 (d)
Develop alternative strategies for change

INTEGRATED MULTI-DISCIPLINARY STRATEGY DEVELOPMENT

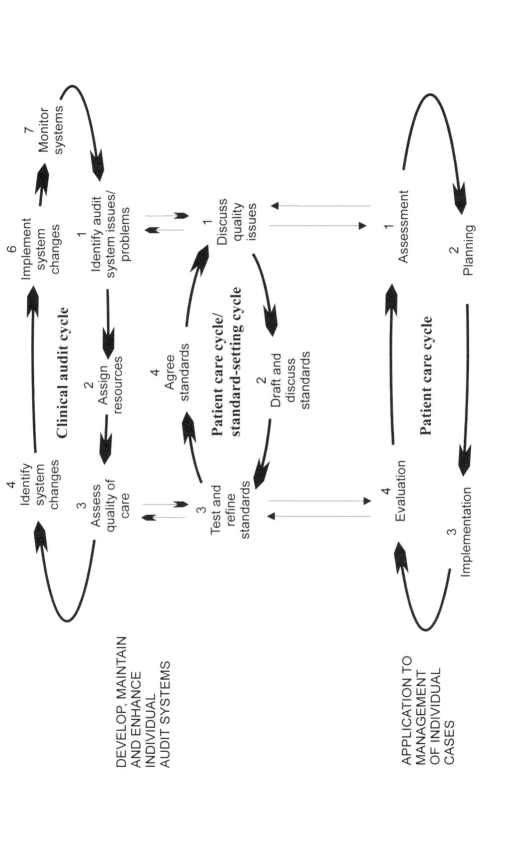

Clinical audit cycle

7 Monitor systems

6 Implement system changes

1 Identify audit system issues/ problems

2 Assign resources

3 Assess quality of care

4 Identify system changes

DEVELOP, MAINTAIN AND ENHANCE INDIVIDUAL AUDIT SYSTEMS

Patient care cycle/ standard-setting cycle

1 Discuss quality issues

2 Draft and discuss standards

3 Test and refine standards

4 Agree standards

Patient care cycle

1 Assessment

2 Planning

3 Implementation

4 Evaluation

APPLICATION TO MANAGEMENT OF INDIVIDUAL CASES

Looking first at the base of the diagram, we feel that the patient care cycle can actually operate at two levels. The first is concerned with individual cases – for example, when assessing the needs of a particular patient and evaluating the care given against a set standard for a particular condition. In our terms, technical and generic issues of quality are likely to be explicit features here. The second looks more generally at the setting and validating of standards, as a system, in the light of data generated from the first stage.

The results of the patient care cycle feed into the clinical audit cycle, which will assess the requirement for changes in the supporting systems connected directly to the provision of care. Groups of cases will be audited as flows of work over time and the implications for the systems set up to handle them will also be assessed – again, technical quality will feature strongly in any analysis of individual systems. An example of this might be determining an appropriate skills mix for a psychiatric ward and then evaluating how well this had been adhered to over, say, a three-month period.

The next level up will be more concerned with multi-disciplinary and multi-professional issues – in our terms primarily systemic quality issues – where changes in one system may well affect how well other systems work. The latter may well be in other peoples' areas of responsibility. For example, there is no point in an accident and emergency department streamlining the way it handles prospective inpatients if the wards and other supporting areas are not geared up to faster admission procedures. This will, in turn, require collaboration between many different services.

We have added a further tier to the Kogan *et al.* figure to incorporate a national audit cycle, in recognition of our belief that there is a need for more supra-hospital auditing. The organizational audit programme run by the King's Fund and the work being pioneered on benchmarking by the Department of Health are important contributions to this field.

Backward mapping and forward mapping

The final area to be discussed in connection with process improvement is the role of external groups. Our view is that some effort should be made to halt, if not reverse, the tendency to forward-map quality improvement activity (see Chapter 3). Currently, the need for most change is still identified by professional and managerial staff and implemented in a top-down and forward-mapping manner. It is only after changes have been made that patients' and carers' views are sought. Effective audit arrangements under TQM would have to take a good deal more account of the customers' views. Figure 4.5 shows how this should be organized at each of the levels discussed above.

Resourcing TQM

Although all models of TQM assume that investment in higher quality will always pay for itself in time, one should be under no illusions about the initial costs of setting up a TQM programme. Our research showed that the cost for an average multiple-site acute unit could easily reach between £300,000 and £350,000 per year for the first two to three years. This assumes that, as a minimum, one would want to fund a central total quality coordinator, four or five directorate facilitators, medical and other audit arrangements, and a substantial TQM training programme.

In a commercial programme these costs would be offset by savings made through reduction in errors and through increased profits from sales to a growing customer base. One would expect the savings in the NHS to be considerably less – first, because the money does not yet truly follow the patient; second, because total income to the NHS is relatively fixed so it is not possible for all TQM sites to increase their income; and third, because considerable emphasis at all TQM sites has been on improving facilities (often a costly business) rather than a preparedness to tackle significant areas of waste.

It is important, therefore, that means are found to reward departments and teams which save money and other resources through process improvement initiatives. We still see frenetic activity before the end of the financial year when 'spend, spend, spend' is the order of the day. Also, there is little encouragement for staff to save money if it is only going to disappear, in its entirety, back into central funds.

We have previously suggested that a formula needs to be found to enable part of the savings to be kept within the departments concerned, part to go into a common TQM pump-priming fund, and part to return to general funds. (The money staying in the department should be for process improvement purposes, not for individual performance-related pay.) We are not specific about the proportions but one-third to each party would seem reasonable.[1]

A further area of cost, particularly in time and effort if not in actual money, is the substantial contribution that TQM expects education and training to make. It was surprising that the majority of our demonstration sites carried out little or no training beyond some initial two- or three-hour TQM awareness-raising events. The kind of substantial training in TQM tools and techniques which we found in commercial programmes was only taking place at three of our sites – even here, only one site had provided substantial coverage.

Where more substantial training was being undertaken, our observations coincided with the views of participants in those programmes – namely that courses employing a format of two or three hours a week for six to ten weeks, interspersed with practical project work back in the workplace, were seen to be more enjoyable and cost-effective than events which followed a format of two or three full days on TQM.

While many staff enjoyed courses which were multi-disciplinary and multi-level, it was clear that trainers found it difficult to bridge the skills and experience gap between staff who had scientific or other research backgrounds and those who were learning about formal techniques of data collection and analysis for the first time.

There should be more varied events than are usually provided in most

TQM programmes. Multi-disciplinary and multi-level workshops may be a good idea for awareness raising and promotion of the general ideas behind TQM. It might be better, however, to provide detailed tools and techniques training to more homogeneous groups which can focus specifically on their own areas of work. Unlike the normal quantitative methods normally taught in TQM, we believe that different measurement techniques would be appropriate for different levels in the organization, and qualitative methods also have an important part to play (see Chapter 4).

Given our analysis of three components of quality – generic, systemic and technical – we think that measurement methods would vary depending on which component of quality was of interest. Confining the technical skills training for TQM to specific groups would also reduce the variation in skills and previous learning within groups. Once people were back in their work and quality groups it might be appropriate once again to provide courses in multi-level and multi-disciplinary settings to facilitate team-building and cross-functional working. (This is discussed more fully in Chapter 4.)

Longer-term issues

Many staff at our research sites felt insufficient effort had been put into recognizing and rewarding departments or individuals who were leading on quality improvement, though this is held to be a key step in quality improvement programmes. While several of our sites had introduced various small schemes for recognizing and rewarding individual performance – for example, employee of the month awards, quality awareness days, newsletter reports and small recognition budgets – little thought appeared to have been given to the longer-term human resources requirements for successful TQM in the NHS.

For example, little had been done at our research sites on the issue of requisite knowledge, attitude and skills for new staff (although we are aware that work is being done elsewhere in the NHS on this). Similarly, individual performance review at our research sites was not being used to specify personal quality objectives based on customer requirements. If TQM is about meeting agreed customer requirements, then the primary purpose of individual performance review at a TQM site should be assessment and appraisal of performance criteria based on these requirements.

Looking further ahead, successfully integrating TQM into the fabric of an organization would seem to suggest that the ability to meet one's customers' requirements should feature in job descriptions and person specifications, and in recruitment, selection, training, promotion, specialization and performance-related pay systems.

Can orthodox TQM work in the NHS?

Although we are fairly confident that the factors described above are significant predictors of TQM movement, much work still needs to be done.

Identifying the issues is one thing – developing effective solutions to some of the problems we have identified is quite another.

This assumes a new importance as more trusts and directly managed units begin the process of implementing structured improvement programmes. There is still a big gap between the rhetoric of quality in trust documentation and business plans, and the reality of implementing systematic quality improvement programmes based on TQM principles. The suggestions made so far in this chapter assume that sites will continue to implement orthodox models of TQM. If this is so, then perhaps the thoughts outlined above will prove helpful.

We believe, however, that these narrow and somewhat prescriptive approaches do not do justice to the range of skills and expertise in the NHS or to the complexity and variation in the work. To that end we propose in our next section a mixed model of quality assurance. This takes the principles behind TQM and suggests how they might be more appropriately implemented in the NHS.

The Brunel quality model (BQM)

Before proposing our own model, we should ask why, overall, the outcomes of the TQM experiments in the NHS were disappointing. We can identify two main reasons which are relevant to future practice. The NHS TQM experiment was underpinned primarily by commercial models and failed to take sufficient account of the realities of a professionally managed public service. Our analysis of the three elements of quality – technical, generic and systemic – suggests that only a multi-modal approach, which seeks to make the best use of existing strengths, will succeed in making the kind of sustained impact that had been hoped for.

Secondly, the Department of Health faced a paradox difficult to resolve. While it was committed to an eclectic approach, in the best tradition of liberal assumptions about change, it also had a more pragmatic purpose – the need to secure commitment to TQM from the sites in order to achieve the Department's general goals. To have implemented the orthodox models of TQM successfully would have required a single-mindedness and rigour difficult for the Department to secure given its traditional relationships with the provider units. The NHS Executive, too, can drive wide organizational change only when it has a government mandate and is thus able to lay down a formal requirement, as with the Patient's Charter.

To us, however, the more fundamental issue is whether it is possible to propose quality assurance procedures which meet the underlying nature of the health service. In order to meet the realities of work in the NHS, and to ensure that the quality initiatives build upon its strengths, a mixed model of quality and quality assurance is needed. It is to this that we now turn.

Our mixed model still draws on the top-down systemic approaches provided by TQM. At the same time it harnesses the expertise available within the NHS, particularly in relation to professional staff. It respects internal differences between disciplines but is equally intended to reorient the organization towards continuous improvement based on users' requirements.

The main features of our mixed model of quality assurance

The main features of our model of quality assurance are

- leadership styles;
- concepts and structures;
- quality definitions and issues of process improvement.

Leadership

Table 8.2 displays the leadership patterns associated with the three approaches to quality assurance – the traditional NHS approach, orthodox TQM and our mixed model. The mixed model (BQM) seeks to provide leadership based on requirements of the task. It would be more

Table 8.2   General features of three approaches to quality assurance

	Orthodox or ideal-typical TQM	*Mixed model*	*Traditional approach*
Leadership of change	Top-down and management-led, supported by specialist quality staff	More even, multi-modal leadership determined by needs. Supported by specialist quality staff	Led by professions supported by administrators. Quality in hands of professionals and administrators
Modes of senior management action (including clinicians)	Evangelistic about single model of quality improvement. Strongly managerial. Looking to reduce variation in definitions of quality. Not empathetic to existing high quality in technical systems	Determined about three elements of quality. Looking to encourage advances in each, having regard to starting points. Support and enable development of local systems with in broader organizational requirement for quality systems. Handle tensions between individual variation and systemic prescription. Role is developmental and multi-modal. Able to move across boundaries	Doctors require other services and groups to orient services to their needs. Professional requirements form basis of quality

even-handed and multi-modal than the other two styles. It advances the need to develop effective quality assurance systems in each function or service. While it requires that the three forms of quality – generic, systemic and technical – are assured through a QA system, the model would allow for negotiation about the priorities and standards set for each area.

Concepts and structures for quality and change
Table 8.3 gives more details about the concepts of structure that underpin the mixed model. Corporate planning would be 'synoptic' or comprehensive as far as the general direction for QA was concerned. In particular, it would emphasize development of an open learning organization committed to individual critical self-reflection and a preparedness to evaluate progress on implementation of QA, as well as the results of monitoring service delivery. Planning for services would be devolved as at present, and development of quality improvement projects would be more opportunistic and incremental than implied by TQM.

As Table 8.3 suggests, there would be some structural differences in the management of quality. The mixed model assumes that quality should be in the hands of line managers. Quality staff would be located in directorates but confined to staff and coordination roles with a specific role to support evaluation.

Concepts of quality
The quality assurance approaches and definitions of quality would be quite different in the three models, as would some of the emphasis on improvement. Table 8.4 outlines some of the key differences. The main features of the mixed model would be the multiple definitions of quality, individually negotiated at service level. These would include generic, systemic and technical components (though with different priorities depending on the nature of the service and an evaluation of current quality levels) and also the needs of different stakeholders. Wherever possible the focus would be on the end users' needs.

The centre would be primarily concerned with working with services to develop effective methods of quality assurance. Standards for generic and systemic quality would be negotiated between the centre and the services, but subject to 'meta-evaluation' by the centre. That is to say, the centre would ensure that services evaluated themselves. QA criteria for individual technical issues would be set by technical services.

However, technical quality would be for negotiation between the service and the centre in conjunction with purchasers where relevant. An important extension might be that the purchaser would work with both parties to develop mutually acceptable QA systems. The purchaser could then evaluate the effectiveness of these systems as an external evaluator. This would be less resource-intensive and more cost-effective than purchasers trying to monitor the quality of individual episodes of care in all the different services. Requirements for QA would form part of purchasers' contracts.

Table 8.3 Concepts and structures in the three approaches

	Orthodox or ideal-typical TQM	Mixed model	Traditional approach
Centre-periphery relationships	Centre leading by example. Each level implements similar predetermined sequence of change	Centre requires services to implement quality systems but allows for variability in design of systems for each function or service	Clear separation based on functional and specialist orientation
Mode of implementation	Top-down cascade of all in planning followed later by bottom-up process improvement	Iterative and helical style. Multi-modal corporate planning – some synoptic/prescriptive, but also more incremental and developmental	Incremental approach to change. Typically focused on input management and technical innovation
Concepts of change	Coercive-prescriptive but with elements of normative re-educative	Mainly normative re-educative. Prescription would be last resort	Self-directed. Diffuse. May start at any level. External direction is high
Structural differences	Start with separate quality meetings structure for quality and normal ongoing business. Facilitators at centre and in units have staff and monitoring roles. In harder models also take on quasi-management responsibilities for change and quality improvement projects	Majority of quality improvement effort would come from line managers, supported by strictly staff role of facilitators located in services. No separate meetings structure, but there would be central quality person with evaluation skills and brief	Quality predominantly in hands of doctors and nursing staff and organized strictly on hierarchical and functional specialist lines. Quality staff, if any, would be confined to patient relations

Table 8.4 Quality definitions and issues of process improvement

	Orthodox or ideal-typical TQM	Mixed model	Traditional approach
Quality assurance approaches	Specialists required to conform to single definition of quality which is driven by customers' requirements	Centre requires periphery to assure quality against a range of central, service and external criteria	Specialists drive definition of quality. QA is primarily by peer review in specialist groupings. Administrators confined to review of administrative systems
Overall definitions of quality	Single definition of 'consistently meeting agreed customer requirements'. Same definition applied to generic, systemic and technical quality. Highly systemic. Seeks to apply systemic to generic and technical quality issue	Multiple definitions but with similar key elements. Balance and content of generic, systemic and technical quality determined by services Key variables might be customer, professional and management quality. Generic and systemic might be weaker than technical	High on technicity for professions and mixture of personal/generic and technical for non-professional staff. Administration, perhaps, more systemic than others. Organizational development led by technical requirements of specialists. Administrators and support services gear themselves to meeting specialist needs, not external customers' needs
Cross-functional process improvement	High cross-functional focus, e.g. business process improvement and re-engineering, all driven by perception of best way to meet customer requirements	Moderate focus on cross-functional activity but always starting from the particular base	Functional specialization. Low cross-functional activity – mainly reactive and demand-led

Other elements of the model
Table 8.5 brings together some of the other factors that make up the three approaches to process improvement. As far as the mixed model is concerned, performance review would feature strongly at both the individual and organizational levels. Both are based on the idea of a self-evaluating organization. Continuous monitoring would feature more strongly than the set-piece audit arrangements most common in the traditional approach and in the way TQM has been implemented so far in much of the NHS.

Evaluation would be directed towards development rather than assessment or appraisal. Due recognition would be given to the limitations that systems place on individual initiative and the emphasis would be on creating the conditions under which individuals could make fuller contributions. The mixed model would draw on the same sort of measurement tools provided for under TQM, though it might employ a wider range of qualitative techniques.

As suggested by the model so far, education and training would be driven by training needs analyses conducted at the base of the organization, not by the kinds of predetermined cascade models to be found under TQM.

An important difference between the three models would be the approach taken to users. Our evaluation of commercial TQM, and the majority of work at NHS TQM sites, suggests that there is little actual empowerment of users although there is no doubt that TQM results in an increased focus on recipients of services.

The mixed model would set out to involve users in the design and evaluation of services, not just in *post hoc* evaluations of satisfaction. The development of informed user groups as evaluators would be a key theme here (see Chapter 4). The issue of backward mapping of service needs and the idea of tapping into the requirements of external groups at different levels are also relevant.

Installing the mixed model

A mixed model would emphasize that the centre helps individual services to develop QA systems for their own use, based on the stages already reached rather than on common definitions of technical or systemic quality. While there would be equal insistence that each unit, department and specialty must implement an explicit QA system, its substantive content would be a matter for local discretion.

There would be a strong emphasis on developing an open learning system but made explicit and firm by the intention to monitor and evaluate the quality of services. This has something in common with the concepts behind the Deming approach in that a more detailed understanding of the characteristics of different processes would be required before attempting to modify them.

The support that each department or discipline needs is different. Pathology, for example, already has a strong tradition of quality control with considerable internal and external validation. However, some services still do not have a good understanding of the differences between quality control, with its stress on identifying and correcting errors, and quality assurance, which is more about designing out errors by systematic attention to the design of processes.

Further, the main technical departments would need support and guidance about how to move from what are currently concerns with technical quality, to issues of generic and systemic quality. There is, however, a base of evaluation expertise in them which can be tapped when seeking such a move.

Some other departments will start from a lower base in technical competence for QA. A new catering service, for example, may need guidance about how to move from a generic concern with customer needs to a more formal technical assurance system, as in a BS 5750 registration. A portering service, trying to improve the transport of patients from wards to theatres, may need help in tackling substantive systemic and cross-functional process improvement issues.

Table 8.5 Performance and training issues in the three models.

	Orthodox or ideal-typical TQM	*Mixed model*	*Traditional approach*
Organization/ department performance review	Diagnostics and benchmarking characterized by comprehensive blanket coverage – staff, purchasers, users, etc.	Diagnostics/ benchmarking more targeted and specific. Issue, thematic, heuristically based. Customers' requirements would also figure strongly but be mediated by professional and process concerns. Development of performance indicators would be by identifying the contribution made by knowledge, values and skills of each group towards achievement of requirements. Harnessing skills would be the overriding concern.	Mainly by peer review for professions. Efficiency of input management and admin processes by administrators. Largely professional criteria but little personal review actually takes place except in cases of negligence. Some IPR now for nurses and administrative staff but still quite rudimentary
Individual performance review	Individual performance (e.g. IPRs) and departmental reviews (e.g. all forms of audit) driven by single factor – that of customers' requirements		

Table 8.5   (Cont.)

	Orthodox or ideal-typical TQM	Mixed model	Traditional approach
Education and training	Distinguishes between education (culture change) and training (tools and techniques for process improvement) Top dictates single definition of quality. All are then trained on top-down basis in approved definition and selected tools Training for quality also seen as separate from, but coordinated with, other forms of training	Sees education as a re-educative, starting from where people are and building on their current knowledge, values and skills. Top dictates requirement for quality assurance systems then engages in meta-evaluation Training would be based on a personal development approach in which quality, including tools and techniques training, would be built into all courses. Emphasis would be on developing open learning approach with strong element of monitoring and evaluation building on what was already available at the base	Professional education is uni-disciplinary and based on technical and formal knowledge. Experts not seen to be competent beyond their specialism (e.g. see Schön, 1983) Medical profession sees education as a means for equipping technical experts with body of esoteric knowledge. Administration sees education as training in general, transferable, administrative skills. Other areas often see training as a matter of learning on the job.
Customer (i.e. patient and external stakeholder) focus	Strongly geared to informing patients and collecting information about their requirements Similar picture to commercial implementations. Customer focus but not empowerment.	Open management which seeks to empower staff and users. But problem of technical jargon and technical nature of QA may make it difficult for them to contribute. Notion of informed user groups may be relevant here	Definitions of need are based on technical and professional views. Users are excluded from the evaluation process as not having the technical competence to contribute.

As to tactics for implementation, we have observed that all departments collect data of some sort. They can be encouraged to do this more systematically and then to begin to question the variations in performance that arise out of existing data. By demonstrating the utility of this approach to quality improvement, it should be possible to encourage them to widen the information base by documenting and analysing more areas of their work. This also has the advantage that they do not start off with a 'problem' – we have noted in both commercial and NHS locations that this can encourage a problem-oriented culture where staff only analyse processes and make changes when there is a problem.

Hunting out obvious problems, particularly when participants come back from their training, sounds efficient but should be seen in the wider context of understanding the processes within which the problems occur. There are many instances of introducing changes without a full consideration of the impact on other internal 'customers' or on the patients or clients.

These are mainly considerations of systemic quality. One should not ignore the opportunity, too, for collaboration on generic quality issues. Much unnecessary effort is expended in organizations in trying to clarify work which has been inadequately prepared, or in chasing up things which have been promised but fail to arrive. Our observations of poor generic quality at several sites suggest that much needs to be done. Tackling generic issues has the advantage that those most concerned with service delivery can at least agree on common definitions of the problems, even if there are disagreements about potential solutions.

In this way staff at all levels get used to cooperating and building up trusting working relationships. One could then move on to systemic and technical quality matters. Although this is an incremental approach it need not necessarily take a lot more time than a drastic top-down and wide-scale approach. Further, time invested at this stage could well be made up with faster progress in later tasks.

Procedures

Those responsible for developing quality must make a choice between TQM and the mixed model described above. If the orthodox TQM model is chosen, this will have the advantage of requiring the use of quite powerful analytical tools and frameworks. A predetermined implementation sequence also allows staff to see what is to happen in the future. Some of our respondents were attracted to the predictability and precision of, for example, the Crosby model.

Such models have the disadvantage, however, of disaggregating elements of process, and the emphasis on a predictable logic of implementation can constrain more creative use of opportunities as they arise. TQM systems also have a 'hardness' of style. Most important, TQM does not build upon existing expertise and is not particularly respectful of professional and other values. It has a value system and logical structure of its own.

The mixed model runs into the danger of 'softness' inasmuch as it deliberately mandates the operating elements of an organization to analyse their own needs and processes for initiating quality, albeit within the policy established by a trust or other unit. Many of the weaker attempts at TQM seen in our study would claim to be filling this prescription. But we suggest a quite rigorous regime for the mixed approach. Simply permitting, or even encouraging, quality developments at the base would not suffice to create a full mixed-model system.

Unlike TQM, it must develop its own working concepts and procedures, although the very process of generating these will itself invite work on, and ownership of, quality generating processes. It has the advantage of reducing conflict between well-established technical and professional concepts of quality, and the more recent focus on quality related to customer requirements. Differentiating *technical* approaches to quality from *systemic* and *generic* elements provides a powerful mechanism for reinforcing the need for broader approaches to quality assurance.

The mixed model will require individual role-holders to operate in multiple modes. They must attend to specialist concepts of quality, and demonstrate to the system that they are evaluating themselves and assuring quality, at the same time as they respond to the whole organization's generic quality policies and policies that ensure that the whole organization works as a total system. This requires a high order of managerial skills (on behalf of managers and clinicians).

Structures

In either system, the leadership of a trust – its chief executive and directors – will head the quality system in stating policies, creating organization and allocating resources to it. The lines of management will then be accountable for installing and carrying through quality procedures. We envisage, however, particularly during the period of installation, that there will be a shadow structure concentrating on quality issues. The shadow structure will be facilitated by a quality director, manager or facilitator, whose primary role will be to assist both management and those working within the operating departments to achieve the quality criteria. In our experience, too, well-selected consultants have made useful inputs.

We envisage the shadow structure as working within a management-led system of regular meetings. The agenda for the meetings should not be merely 'educational' but should have substance. A typical agenda for a meeting might include all or some of the following items:

(a) receiving reports on the ways in which departments are working within the three modes of quality assurance (technical, generic and systemic);
(b) encouraging and receiving reports on specific quality projects;

(c) deciding how the total organization can better facilitate (a) and (b);
(d) ensuring linkage with other quality initiatives (such as the Patient's Charter, contractual procedures, or different forms of audit);
(e) identifying training needs and authorizing provision of training for quality;
(f) supporting the operational units in self-evaluation of their quality initiatives – this leaves aside the question of how the organization will evaluate and monitor the initiatives: we will return to this later.

Training

Training needs should be identified collaboratively between the managers of departments and the quality facilitators, using the shadow quality structure. The starting point should be local conceptions of quality needs. In identifying needs the quality facilitators should be rigorous and eclectic. They should not, for example, throw overboard some of the valuable TQM concepts and techniques, particularly those concerned with data collection and measurement. They should also work with the operational departments on the elusive question of outcomes.

Resourcing

It is implicit in the mixed model that quality development should start with the operational departments and that quality resources should form part of their budgets. Central resourcing will be necessary, however, for the provision of the quality facilitators and for across-the-board training and publicity. It is unlikely that the mixed model will be any more or less expensive than a TQM model.

Evaluation

A TQM model assumes that evaluation will be in the hands of the central entity and that it will evaluate against preset criteria determined by the model itself. A mixed model assumes that the central entity will be concerned with installing and implementing generic and systemic concepts of quality and will, therefore, be evaluating its own efforts and those of the operating departments in these respects. It would set criteria for evaluation of progress on the implementation of QA. Choice of criteria and standards for systemic and generic quality would be a matter for negotiation between the centre and the services.

As far as specialist working is concerned, however, it will be for the operational departments to evaluate themselves, but to make manifest to the central organization that they are doing so. The function of the centre will therefore be one of meta-evaluation.

Conclusion

Those embarking on quality assurance have a hard row to hoe. It requires efforts that are both intellectual and organizational, or even political. Any of the variants of TQM that we have noted or proposed involves a culture change in organizations whose strength has largely depended on multiple cultures and knowledge systems.

It is therefore important that the need for change is convincingly identified and generally accepted, and that can only happen if good diagnostic work on shortfalls in quality is undertaken. There then has to be consensus about the nature of the changes needed, and this involves shared understanding of the nature of quality and what might stand in its way. And then there has to be commitment to procedures and structures for change.

We hope that we have shown the way in which these problems can be tackled without disguising the difficulties to be faced in doing so.

Note

1 See also the Audit Commission's (1992) observations on the general issues of promoting and sustaining QA systems in the NHS. The Commission potentially has a significant part to play through shifting the focus on audits to support changes in handling

Appendix 1
Comparison of the integration of some Department of Health initiatives

TQM objectives	Patient's Charter	Resource Management Initiative	Medical audit	Compulsory competitive tendering
1 Customers' definitions of need put at centre of process improvement	Not directly – waiting times *are* a patient concern but standards are not set locally in response to local customer requirements as would be required under TQM	Not a strong feature, although some link to internal customers. Presumptions of indirect indirect link to patient care	Not in standard medical audit, though there are a few examples of audit which specifically build in patients' views	Not a feature. Internal and external customers rarely consulted about their requirements prior to tender. Also problem of single supplier relationships
2 Collective definitions of quality across whole organization	No actual definition of quality. Also many parts of service not involved in Charter	Not designed to achieve this	Yes, at least between doctors, but does not include nurses or support services, etc.	Does not produce common definitions but quality likely to be specified in contracts
3 Reductions in inter-disciplinary barriers	Has potential to achieve these through limited multi-disciplinary collaboration – e.g. over waiting times	Should achieve these because those responsible for own activity must consult others involved in process management	Yes, within and between specialties but not between doctors and other staff	No *a priori* reason why CCT should produce this. Opposite could be the case where ownership of quality is low

TQM objectives	Patient's Charter	Resource Management Initiative	Medical audit	Compulsory competitive tendering
4 Reductions in errors and waste	Not directly, but might achieve these indirectly through analysis of processes	Definitely should result in savings. More likely to be savings in waste than in errors	Yes, especially where local medical audit includes use of resources. More likely to result in savings in errors than in waste	May lead to this but not always without compromising other aspects of quality
5 'Obsessive' commitment to continuous quality improvement	Not a specified objective – standards in this format are relatively static and emphasize minimum performance	Yes, but only in respect of optimum use of resources – not in patient satisfaction	Yes, in respect of technical and professional quality but not designed to enhance overall quality of patient experience	Not likely to result – but there will almost certainly be a commitment to monitoring existing standards in contracts
6 Major commitment to training and education in quality improvement techniques	No training for staff specified	Yes, in relation to use of management information, but not in use of specific process improvement tools	Yes, in that it is a vehicle for education, but only weakly related to existing medical training and weaker still to quality improvement techniques	Few contracts specify training and development requirements other than national minimum standards – no training in quality improvement
7 Provision of enhanced management information	Could lead to better management information if performance is monitored on an ongoing basis	Definitely – the prime purpose of the initiative	In theory, yes, *providing* general aggregated information is made available to management	Yes – monitoring of contract specifications will provide useful management information

Appendix II
Selected reading on evaluation and measurement

These are some of the more easily available texts on evaluation, social research methods and measurement techniques. They are included because we think they would be helpful to people working in the area of evaluation of quality. We have organized them under different headings and so some texts appear more than once.

Evaluation and research methods

CEPPP (1992) *Considering Quality: An Analytical Guide to the Literature on Quality and Standards in the Public Services*. Centre for the Evaluation of Public Policy and Practice, Brunel University, London.
   An overview of some of the more important literature on quality and evaluations of quality in the private sector, health care, education, social security, local government services, housing management and the police service. Also contains a brief but worthwhile discussion of issues surrounding the definition of quality.
Jick, T. (1983) 'Mixing qualitative and quantitative methods: triangulation in action' in J. Van Maanen (ed.), *Qualitative Methodology*. Sage Publications Ltd, London.
   For those who want to rely mainly on quantitative methods, this is an interesting discussion of triangulation. Again, those with a deeper interest in qualitative research techniques would do well to look at the whole book.
Light, D. (1983) 'Surface data and deep structure: observing the organisation of professional training' in J. Van Maanen (ed.), *Qualitative Methodology*. Sage Publications Ltd, London.
   An extremely interesting and insightful set of observations on training. Should be required reading for those who are strong believers in quantitative methods of measurement for human processes. The chapter is key to understanding how observation and observational techniques can aid our analysis of human process.
Tudiver, F., Bass, M., Dunn, E., Norton, P. and Stewart, M. (1992) *Assessing*

Interventions: Traditional and Innovative Methods, Research Methods for Primary Care, Volume IV. Sage Publications Ltd, London.
A useful introduction to different methods of evaluation in primary care. Looks at qualitative and quantitative techniques. Of wider interest than just primary care. Good examples of actual studies.

The following suggestions describe different techniques and cover particularly well the limitations and pitfalls of different approaches:

Ackroyd, S. and Hughes, J. A. (1981) *Data Collection in Context.* Longman, Harlow.
Blalock, A. B. and Blalock, H. M. (1982) *Introduction to Social Research,* Prentice Hall, Englewood Cliffs, New Jersey.
Shipman, M. (1981) *The Limitations of Social Research.* Longman, Harlow.

Evaluations of quality, TQM, audit, etc.

Henkel, M. (1991) *Government, Evaluation and Change.* Jessica Kingsley Publishers, London.
Two excellent chapters for the serious/advanced reader. The first covers an earlier classic evaluation by M. Henkel, M. Kogan, T. Packwood, P. Whitaker and P. Youll (1989), *The Health Advisory Service: An Evaluation.* King Edward's Hospital Fund, London. The second chapter is an elegant discussion on evaluative models, methods and knowledge. Other chapters would also be of value to those with a deeper interest in evaluation.
Kerrison, S., Packwood, T. and Buxton, M. (1993) *Medical Audit: Taking Stock,* Medical Audit Series, Number 6, Brunel University Health Economics Research Group and King's Fund Centre. Published by King's Fund Centre, London.
Essential reading for anyone concerned with setting up or evaluating medical audit. The authors' evaluation is based on a case study of the introduction of audit in general medicine at four hospitals. The study also reports the results of a national survey of staff working in medical audit.
Kogan, M., Redfern, S., Kober, A., Norman, I., Packwood, T. and Robinson, S. (1995) *Clinical Audit in Four Health Professions.* Joint Report by the Centre for the Evaluation of Public Policy and Practice, Brunel University, and the Nursing Research Unit, King's College, London University.
A detailed analysis of clinical audit in clinical psychology, occupational therapy, physiotherapy and speech and language therapy, following on the Normand Report. Particularly important are the sections on analysis and modelling of audit cycle (Chapters 6 and 12) – copies are available from the Nursing Research Unit at King's College, London. Also available from autumn 1995 by the same authors, *Making Use of Clinical Audit.* Open University Press.
Macdonald, J. (1993), *TQM: Does It Always Work?,* TQM Practitioners Series. Technical Communications Publishing Ltd, Letchworth.
Macdonald, co-author of the excellent *Global Quality – the New Management Culture* (see below), discusses some of the major reasons why TQM programmes fail. This is one of the few works to analyse the difficulties in implementing TQM. It covers weaknesses in Western understanding of TQM, the lack of management commitment, the lack of planning, over-reliance on TQM tools, a critique of Crosby, the issue of top-down versus bottom-up, and the lack of proper measurement. Well worth reading.

Pfeffer, N. and Coote, A. (1991) *Is Quality Good for You? – A Critical Review of Quality Assurance in Welfare Services*. Institute for Public Policy Research, London.

An excellent monograph charting the developments in quality of the last 100 years and presenting a new 'democratic' model of quality for welfare services. This should be on anyone's shortlist of books on quality in the public sector.

Portsmouth Hospitals Pharmaceutical Service (1993) *Progress on Quality Management of Pharmaceutical Services*. Portsmouth Hospitals Pharmacy Staff, Portsmouth Hospitals, Portsmouth.

This is one of the few units where we have seen ISO 9004 being well implemented within a wider quality management programme and contextualized for hospital services. This is the third of the progress reports and contains a wealth of detail on the progress made on a number of different measures for ward services, inpatients and outpatients supplies, community health unit service, and so on. It would be very helpful to anyone charged with implementing ISO 9004 or BS 5750 in hospital services.

TQM – 'how to do it' books

Edvardsson, B., Thomasson, B. and Øvretveit, J. (1994) *Quality of Service: Making it Really Work*. McGraw-Hill Book Company Europe, Maidenhead.

A good introductory chapter to quality measurement, contrasting quantitative and qualitative methods and covering the SERVQUAL scale. More detailed descriptions of SERVQUAL are available in Zeithaml *et al.* (1990) and Babbakus and Mangold (1992) (see next section).

Koch, H. (1991) *Total Quality Management in Health Care*. Longman Group UK Ltd, Harlow.

An expensive, but excellent, 'how to do it' book on TQM. Covers preparation for TQM, organization and management, standard setting, clinical audit, communications and training.

Oakland, J. (1989) *Total Quality Management*. Heinemann Professional Publishing, Oxford.

Justifiably one of the standard texts on TQM. Particularly good on measurement, including an introduction to statistical process control. Biased towards the private sector. Draws little on other organizational literature.

Øvretveit, J. (1992) *Health Service Quality: An Introduction to Quality Methods for Health Services*. Blackwell Scientific Publications, Oxford.

An excellent discussion of quality methods, pointing out that there are different issues when considering client quality, professional quality and management quality. These may well require different methods of measurement. Appendix III also gives details of the MAPS-QUAL method for formulating quality strategies. The method is based on the Malcum Baldridge National Quality Award criteria. The book is essential reading for anyone with responsibility for quality improvements in the NHS.

Measurement and measurement techniques

Babbakus, E. and Mangold, W. (1992) 'Adapting the SERVQUAL scale to hospital services: an empirical investigation', *Health Services Research,* vol. 26, no. 6, February. A good account of applying SERVQUAL in a health environment.

Banaka, W. H. (1971) *Training in In-Depth Interviewing*. Harper & Row, New York.

If you are going to use unstructured interview techniques to get at qualitative data, and still want to end up with reliable results at the end of the process, then this book is well worth reading.

Department of Health (1993) *Monitoring Made Easy*. BAPS Health Publications Unit, Haywood, Lancashire.

Produced in association with the NHS Training Directorate, this is an excellent guide to basic measurement techniques, including questionnaires, interviews, observational studies, and the use of mystery shoppers. The text covers the pitfalls of sampling, how to analyse data and effective presentation. It includes a number of exercises, with the answers. It is based around the Patient's Charter, and more detailed technical guidance in a similar vein is available from the Patient's Charter Unit in Leeds.

Edvardsson, B., Thomasson, B. and Øvretveit, J. (1994) *Quality of Service: Making it Really Work*. McGraw-Hill Book Company Europe, Maidenhead.

A good introductory chapter to quality measurement, contrasting quantitative and qualitative methods and covering the SERVQUAL scale. More detailed descriptions of SERVQUAL are available in Zeithaml *et al.* (1990) and Babbakus and Mangold (1992).

Graham, I. (1992) *TQM in Service Industries*, TQM Practitioners Series. Technical Communications Publishing Ltd, Letchworth.

A strong supporter of the Deming approach, Graham has produced an excellent introduction to the use of flow-charting, cause–effect analysis, and a detailed application in a case study based on a ferry company.

MacIver, S. (1991) *Obtaining the Views of Outpatients*. Quality Improvement Programme, King's Fund Centre, London.

This booklet and others in the series, including one on inpatients and one on mental health patients, is well worth a look by those charged with designing patient satisfaction measures.

Neave, H. (1990) *The Deming Dimension*. SPC Press Inc., Knoxville, TN.

The definitive interpretation of Deming's approach to quality improvement. Not very well written, and rather sycophantic, but the description of variation and control of processes, including Deming's experiments, is one of the best there is. It includes a detailed discussion of Deming's 14 points.

Oakland, J. (1989) *Total Quality Management*. Heinemann Professional Publishing, Oxford.

Justifiably one of the standard texts on TQM. Particularly good on measurement, including an introduction to statistical process control. Biased towards the private sector. Draws little on other organizational literature.

Øvretveit, J. (1992) *Health Service Quality: An Introduction to Quality Methods for Health Services*. Blackwell Scientific Publications, Oxford.

An excellent discussion of quality methods, pointing out that there are different issues when considering client quality, professional quality and management quality. These may well require different methods of measurement. Appendix III also gives details of the MAPS-QUAL method for formulating quality strategies. The method is based on the Malcum Baldrige National Quality Award criteria. The book is essential reading for anyone with responsibility for quality improvements in the NHS.

Randall, L. and Senior, M. (1992) *Managing and Improving Quality and*

Delivery. TQM Practitioners Series, Technical Communications Publishing Ltd, Letchworth.
An excellent discussion of the differences between customers' and employees' views of service quality and how to align the two. Two commercial service case studies are worth looking at for the identification of service attributes. In particular, one refers to hospital hotel services. A good basic introduction to designing, implementing and analysing questionnaires.

Rosander, A. (1989) *The Quest for Quality in Services*, Quality Resources. The Kraus Organisation Ltd, White Plains, NY.
An authoritative look at statistical techniques with a wealth of worked examples and case studies. Of particular interest for the health service is Rosander's discussion about customers being 'a sample of one'. See particularly pages 503–13, in which he shows the fallacy of applying statistical techniques to patient quality. As he says: 'A sick person desiring medical service is a sample of one. There is no mean, no variance, no distribution. It is not a statistical problem. It is a medical problem although . . . statistics may be applied to medical research.'

Roundtree, D. (1991) *Statistics without Tears: A Primer for Non-mathematicians*. Penguin Books, London.
This is an excellent easy introduction to statistics and could be valuable to anyone starting out on analysing data for the first time.

United Bristol Hospital Healthcare Trust (1991) *Patient Survey Unit: Outline and Philosophy*. UBHCT and Bristol Royal Infirmary, Bristol.
Overall, we were very disappointed with the examples of patient satisfaction questionnaires we saw during our research (though things were getting better by late 1993). However, this excellent patient survey unit, set up by Bette Baldwin and others, demonstrates that high-quality measures can be designed to test customer responsiveness within a broad, well-thought-out ethical framework. This booklet outlines the philosophy of the unit which can also be approached for examples of a wide range of well-designed questionnaires.

Wheeler, D. and Chambers, D. (1990) *Understanding Statistical Process Control*. Addison-Wesley, Wokingham.
A detailed and heavyweight text book on SPC. Full of good examples on different techniques for describing variation, using descriptive statistics, control charts and attribute data. If you have to get into SPC, this is one of the more readable books.

Zeithaml, V., Parasuraman, A. and Berry, L. (1990) *Delivering Quality Service – Balancing Customer Perceptions and Expectations*. The Free Press, New York.
A detailed description of the design and use of the SERVQUAL measure.

Trends in evaluation, quality, health services

Harrison, S. and Pollitt, C. (1994) *Controlling Health Professionals – The Future of Work and Organization in the NHS*. Open University Press, Buckingham.
A timely and well-argued analysis of the changing nature of the NHS and its professional staff. Good sections on quality in health care and the implications of new definitions of quality for professionals and other staff.

Henkel, M. (1991) *Government, Evaluation and Change*. Jessica Kingsley Publishers, London.
Two excellent chapters for the serious/advanced reader. The first covers an earlier classic evaluation by M. Henkel, M. Kogan, T. Packwood, P. Whitaker and

P. Youll (1989) *The Health Advisory Service: An Evaluation.* King Edward's Hospital Fund, London. The second chapter is an elegant discussion on evaluative models, methods and knowledge. Other chapters would also be of value to those with a deeper interest in evaluation.

Hoggett, P. (1991) 'A new management in the public sector?', *Policy and Politics*, vol. 19, No. 4, October.
An excellent paper reviewing progress in public sector management where centralized, bureaucratic modes of organization are giving way to operational decentralization.

Macdonald, J. and Piggott, J. (1990) *Global Quality – The New Management Culture.* Mercury Books, London.
The authors have been pioneers in much of the development of TQM ideas and also have a good track record of implementing TQM in (mainly) commercial environments. Well worth reading for its summary of the ideas of Crosby, Deming, Juran and other 'gurus'.

Sanderson, I. (ed.) (1992) *Management of Quality in Local Government.* Local Economic and Social Strategy Series, Longman Group UK, Harlow.
Although health care is only discussed in passing, there are good chapters on defining quality in a local government context, managing the issue of decentralization, and improving quality by research. There is also an excellent discussion of quality in the context of the 'New Right', the 'New Left' and 'New Managerialism' by John Bermington and Matthew Taylor in the same book.

Appendix III
Criteria used to evaluate TQM at the NHS TQM pilot sites

The following extract is taken from Joss *et al.* (1991, pp. 46–9):

18 Following our decision to evaluate criteria based on outcomes at each of the input, process and output stages, we list below the outcomes we looked for from each stage:

Outcomes of changes in inputs

19 Context, conceptualization and programme objective outcomes:

    (a) an improved understanding by staff at the site of the context faced by the Department of Health and its rationale for introducing TQM

    (b) benchmarks derived from an analysis of the context facing the site – in particular, what were the existing quality states and concepts of quality at that time; also what data was collected on staff and customer views

    (c) the resulting objectives of TQM as expressed within projects

    (d) an understanding about different models of organizational change and of available models of TQM; construction of a coherent model

    (e) the development of mission statements, value statements, aims, goals, objectives, targets and plans which are consistent with stated aims of TQM and which are internally consistent and coherent

    (f) strategies for securing staff commitment, development and behavioural change

In addition we are also interested in the more general issues of:

    (g) the rationale behind the Department's choice of TQM as a vehicle for change

    (h) the resulting objectives of TQM as established by the Department of Health

    (i) what models of change were implicit in the different projects and their assumptions about future working of NHS systems.

20 Outcomes from a review of structure

One might expect a TQM site to develop a structure which promoted:

(a) the opportunity for corporate decision-making, especially about quality issues
(b) a reduction in barriers between different functions and groups
(c) improved vertical and lateral communication
(d) explicit vertical and lateral accountability for quality issues throughout the organization, with an integration of responsibility for quality in management and professional roles.

21 Outcomes from a review of resource requirements

The following are held to be four important areas of resourcing:

(a) sufficient resources for the training of all staff (including top management) in order that they are committed to a philosophy of continuous improvement and have the skills to implement it
(b) resources for the development of high quality information for process improvement purposes
(c) skilled resources to provide technical and practical support for monitoring and evaluation activity
(d) we were also interested in whether or not sites had been able to cost the implementation of TQM and, if so, whether this could be set against identifiable savings made through process improvement.

Outcomes of changes in systems and processes

22 The following might be outcomes from changes to, and realignment of, systems and processes:

(a) corporate, functional and departmental level planning for quality improvement
(b) multi-disciplinary activity to improve selected processes
(c) continuous monitoring of performance in all processes
(d) recognition and reward for all staff for their efforts to improve quality in their own areas of work
(e) empowerment of staff and customers to contribute to service-planning, development, delivery and evaluation
(f) enhancement of the quality and availability of information required for process improvement purposes
(g) a sufficient level of training to enable all staff to contribute to continuous improvement within their own processes
(h) establishment of realistic but comprehensive systems for performance review
(j) development of criteria, processes and procedures for evaluation of their projects
(k) integration of previous and new initiatives with TQM.

Again, more generally, we are also interested in

(l) the extent to which the implementation has been put into effect and whether, and by how much, it has slipped from original objectives

(m) the extent to which TQM arrangements display a good level of logic inasmuch as defined activities are well related to the aims attempted

(n) the quality of needs analysis, its relationship to research analysis, service delivery and its capacity to incorporate the end-users' perceptions of their requirements

(p) the training assumptions implicit in TQM objectives, the procedures adopted, and the extent to which TQM has percolated non-TQM training programmes

Outcomes of changes in outputs

23 These might be some of the more important outcomes to result from changed outputs:

(a) a genuinely committed senior management team with an obsession about continuous quality improvement

(b) an organization-wide quality planning system which has achieved a common understanding about definitions of quality and the need for continuous improvement within a given model of TQM

(c) improved information systems which provide both internal and external customers with the information they need to contribute to service-planning, development, delivery and evaluation

(d) empowered consumers who are enabled and encouraged to contribute to improvement in services

(e) empowered staff who have the commitment and skills to contribute to continuous improvement

(f) evidence of reductions in multi-disciplinary barriers and more cooperative multi-disciplinary working

(g) genuine improvements having been achieved in a range of targeted processes

(h) identifiable savings in wastage through getting it right first time; more cost-effective use of resources

(j) increases in internal customer satisfaction with services received within internal customer chains

(k) positive changes in health status of patients; their perception of the quality of information received, and their general satisfaction with the total episode

(l) a reorientation of services offered, on the basis of a more developed understanding of the needs of consumers and other interested stakeholders.

More general issues include the following:

(m) the extent to which the senior management team, if committed to TQM, has managed to sustain respect for the range of professional values

(n) changes that may have occurred in organizational and professional cultures. These would include changes in priorities between different values, shifts from individualistic professional aims towards more holistic aims evincing concern for the whole enterprise in which individuals have a place

(p) changes which may have taken place in assumptions about service delivery in terms of impact on users (internal and external). We hope to build up a model for the study of impacts on end-users though such an analysis will not be applied within this project

(q) the impact of TQM on inter-agency working and on working between different disciplines within the health service

(r) the capacity of the whole organization to learn from the TQM initiatives, internal and external. The creation and use of networks for diffusion and learning.

Numbers and roles of staff interviewed at NHS and commercial sites during evaluation

NHS TQM sites

Roles	1991	1992	% of 1992 interviewees also interviewed in 1991	1993	% of 1993 interviewees also interviewed in 1992	Totals
Admin management[1]	118	36	83	27	59	181
Admin non-management	11	11	56	8	62	30
Support services clinical management	16	19	84	17	53	52
Support services clinical non-management	5	5	80	6	67	16
Support services non-clinical management	11	18	61	11	64	40
Support services non-clinical non-management	6	4	100	7	43	17
Nurse managers	40	16	83	11	82	67
Nurses	38	22	77	15	53	75
Clinical directors	12	6	100	6	67	24
Consultants	9	6	33	11	54	26
GPs	2	–	–	–	–	2
Paramedic managers	18	6	83	6	67	30
Paramedics	2	2	50	3	67	7
CHC members	2	–	–	–	–	2
Totals	290	151	77	128	60	569

[1] Includes quality staff, trainers, personnel, finance and headquarters management staff.
Source: Joss et al. (1994, Chapter 4).

NHS non-TQM sites

Roles	1992	1993	% interviewed in both 1992 and 1993	Total number of interviews
Admin management	17	25	52	42
Admin non-management	13	8	88	21
Clinical management	12	8	75	20
Support services clinical non-management	3	2	100	5
Support services non-clinical management	8	10	70	18
Support services non-clinical non-management	2	1	100	3
Nursing management	8	12	58	20
Nurses	7	11	45	18
Clinical directors	2	4	50	6
Consultants	8	5	62	13
GPs				
Paramedic managers	4	4	100	8
Paramedics	2	1	100	3
CHC/others				0
				0
Totals	86	91	67%[1]	177

[1] Averaged across all roles.
Source: Joss *et al.* (1994, Chapter 5).

Commercial companies

Sites	1992 sample	1993 sample	Number of 1993 interviewees also interviewed in 1992
Thames Water Utilities	32	27	15 (55%)
Post Office Counters	22	23	12 (57%)
Totals	54	50	

Source: Joss *et al.* (1994, Chapter 6).

Appendix V
The phenomenon of convergence at the commercial sites

Post Office Counters

Int. process chains	Short – many lateral relationships
Company history	Fairly clear; national network; single employer; new chairman ex-Xerox
Working processes	Well understood and well documented. Relatively small variation except in some local processes
Customer base	Increasingly volatile base with more alternatives for customers – e.g. banks building socs, retail chains
Previous QI approaches	Little in way of structured or comprehensive approaches to QI
Product/ service range	Wide range of products and services – capable of expansion in absolute turnover, market share and diversification

RESPONSES IN YEAR 1 TO INITIAL ANALYSIS

Top-down corporate TQM with full shadow quality meetings' structure

Revolutionary approach

Training-led QIPs

Set-piece QIPs and considerable cross-functional activity

System-driven change

Strong external customer-focus with extensive surveys

Management behaviour feedback system

LOCATIONS CHOSEN BY COMPANIES FOR PILOTING TQM

Headquarters and three pilot TQM sites (districts) out of 30 plus all of HQ

Thames Water Utilities

Int. process chains	Very long with less lateral relationships
Company history	Chequered history with amalgamations of many small and large companies
Working processes	Poorly documented. Considerable variation throughout supply, distribution, sewage treatment, etc.
Customer base	Stable/captive base, but increased pressure from shareholders and EC/government watchdogs
Previous QI approaches	Strong emphasis on QC in water quality control but little experience of QA/TQM approaches in other areas
Product/ service range	Few products and services – i.e. water supply and sewage & sewage treatment. Limited expansion or diversification possible – tension between expansion and conservation

Strong bottom-up decentralized approach. Quality in hands of line managers

Three-stage evolutionary approach:

understanding and documenting processes

process control through systematic measurement

process improvement

Mainly voluntary involvement

Weak links between external customers and internal processes

Almost all developments involved uni-disciplinary and intra-departmental documentation of processes

Weak internal customer links between processes

Thames Quality Awards (now over 700 locations working towards or secured awards)

BS 5750 in Engineering (now achieved)

Two pilot TQM sites (sewage and water treatment works)

| ANALYSIS BY END OF YEAR 2 | RESPONSES TO ANALYSIS OF YEAR 2 | YEAR 3 ?? |

Tension between potential for a problem-oriented culture and QI as normal practice

Strong internal customer links developing – restructuring will help here

Number of highly successful QIPs including cross-functional

Set-piece approach of QIPs did not provide sufficient opportunity for continuous improvement of small-scale processes

High owership if people are involved in QIPs after initial training, but this can fade

Integrating Customer First and Business as Usual

Shift to more overt continuous improvement.

Moving away from formal set-piece QIPs towards larger number of smaller-scale quality improvement activities

Devolving power to periphery and widening involvement of staff

Restructuring to flatten management hierarchy, gain process ownership, and service level agreements

Further convergence

Progress more variable than Post Office Counters – much less training undertaken

Stronger individual ownership in TQAs but less so in BS 5750. Only one of two pilot TQM site showing marked progress

Substantial improvements in process documentation

Weaknesses in personal QI skills becoming evident as Thames Water moves towards process improvement

Need recognized for stronger internal and external customer links

Need for more training and development in tools and techniques for data collection

Centre beginning to apply more quality structure, coordination and direction to business units. More facilitation and expertise provided to support front-line staff

Introducing work flow champions and service level agreements to improve and formalize internal customer chains and build in the end users

Process engineering study to realign central processes and process owners with business needs

Appendix VI

Example of a diagnostic chart for quality in health systems

Organizational levels	Stage reached	Organizational structure	Culture (including leadership)	Systematic measurement	Customer-driven quality
STRATEGIC LEVEL: (Total Quality Management)	High	Fully integrated business and quality planning structure, both laterally and vertically. Head of Quality is main board appointment. Quality Steering Group staffed by board-level members including doctors.	All senior managers/ clinical directors are actively committed to CQI. They act as role models for CQI in behaviour as well as rhetoric. Have produced and promote documented vision, mission, and organizational objectives which integrate quality and business planning.	Strategic planning is driven by backward-mapped internal and external customer data combined with competitor benchmarking. Board demonstrates commitment to systematic measurement by explicitly measuring own performance.	External customers/ informed user groups involved at all levels and stages of service planning including strategic issues of contracting, service prioritization, etc. All HR systems – recruiting, training, etc. – promote/sustain culture of CQI.
Corporate Planning Integrating business and quality planning across total organization	Medium	Formal structure and mechanisms for quality planning present, but still not well linked to normal business planning. Planning driven by costs not quality.	Some key managers and clinical directors committed to and knowledgeable about own TQM initiative but others yet to be convinced. Integrated planning system in early stages – not yet to be fully established.	Effort being made at centre to promote integrated model of data collection, but not yet in place. Good data being collected at each level but forward mapping the dominant mode. Meta-evaluation is weak.	Internal customer chains established with service level agreements in place. External customers not systematically or routinely involved in service planning.

	Low	Lack of structure and mechanisms for strategic quality planning – e.g. no QSG. Business planning not linked to such quality planning as takes place.	Deep divisions exist between perceptions of managers, clinicians and other staff about what TQM approach, if any, to follow. Only rudimentary quality planning system. Financial planning holds sway.	Poor integration of IS/IT. Lack of attention to cross-functional data needs. Culture still one of ready, fire, aim. Many examples of change without data collection/analysis.	Little/no part played by external customers in strategic planning process. Notion of internal customers enters vocabulary but not idea of chains.
DIRECTORATE LEVEL: (cross-functional quality assurance)	High	Fully coordinated and integrated structures for CQI across whole organization. All forms of audit are integrated and follow common structures.	Clinical and other directors put overall good of organization above individual directorate needs. Work flow champions working on cross-functional quality improvement. Business process improvement/re-engineering successfully undertaken.	Systems in place for cross-functional process improvement. Reviews are commonplace. Backward mapping is a distinct feature. Patient-focused care units are well established.	Systematic backward mapping of complete processes has provided for uniformly high, customer-driven, quality across directorate boundaries.

Organizational levels	Stage reached	Organizational structure	Culture (including leadership)	Systematic measurement	Customer-driven quality
Designing/ implementing cross-functional process improvement systems across directorates	Medium	Most departments now linked in common cross-functional approaches within directorates but cross-functional CQI poorly organized *across* directorate boundaries.	In the exploratory stages of improving interface with other departments. Improved cooperation but mainly on a needs basis. Little proactive effort as yet. Specific people being appointed to review interfaces.	Detailed thinking taking place about cross-functional process improvement – e.g. following business process improvement or re-engineering. One or two examples of improvement of larger processes evident.	Departments now well integrated re their joint customers (internal and external) but differences still marked across directorate boundaries.
	Low	Most departments pursuing own models of quality improvement. No directorate level QIG. Poor coordination between departments and directorates.	Directorates work as individual entities. Win-lose situations are common. Tend to blame other departments for poor quality. Little effort to improve interface with others.	Directorates operate as independent units, collaborating infrequently when serious problems arise. Fundamental differences of view about patient care so relevance of data collected is unnecessarily disputed.	Well-developed single systems but customers moving between departments encounter different levels of customer-driven quality.

DEPARTMENTAL LEVEL: (single system quality assurance) Refining/ developing quality assurance systems within a department	High	Fully integrated structure for quality at departmental level including integration with all forms of audit. QIGs highly successful groups. Membership is rotated to give all chance to work on one. Competition for membership.	Considerable collaboration on joint development of approaches to quality. Doctors and managers subscribe to similar basic model of quality and work together to promote shared vision. Both to be found attending training events together on TQM.	Performance of managers is tied directly to what is required from them to meet/exceed customers' expectations. Systematic measurement occurs in all significant processes, not just where there are problems.	Development of new systems driven by customers' views. Many examples of customers systematically involved in design, delivery and evaluation.
	Medium	Formally convened and systematically resourced QIGs. Coordinated objectives across linked to organizational goals. Only one of lateral or vertical structures is well integrated.	All forms of audit are in place but still lack of vertical or lateral integration. Managers and doctors collaborate on a needs basis with one or two proactive developments. Appreciation of each others positions but inter-dependence describes relationships.	Mainly reactive data collection by committed individuals though where happening it is well organized and follows taught model of problem-solving. Much effort going on to spread discipline of systematic data collection and analysis to uncommitted groups.	Good systems for gaining customers' views and for developing services, but links between two still poor.

Organizational levels	Stage reached	Organizational structure	Culture (including leadership)	Systematic measurement	Customer-driven quality
	Low	Informal structure for QIGs. which come and go on voluntary basis. Objectives/ projects not linked to organizational goals. Unsystematically and poorly resourced. Little desire by majority to serve on QIGs or QITs.	Doctors pursuing medical audit unintegrated with other audits. Managers and doctors in constant disagreement with little forward movement, about what constitute appropriate measures of quality.	Systematic measurement confined, in main, to QIGs. Even here there is tendency to cut corners and miss out on pre-test or post-test stages. Over-reliance on unplanned and evaluated change.	Gaining customers' views and involving them in developing own service is at best sporadic. Poor links between views and QA systems development.
TEAM/ SECTION LEVEL: (personal quality improvement) Personal and small group process improvement	High	Common approach to QI. Substantial coordinated quality improvement activity going on fully supported by committed managers/ doctors. Full-time or part-time fully trained facilitators in place.	Majority of staff highly committed to organization's model of TQM. Internal and external customers requirements form the basis for all individual service delivery. Constant effort by individual staff to improve.	Substantial majority of staff involved in some way in collecting data on own and work group's performance. Multiple methods in use. CQI from a user's perspective is a way of life. Not locked into problem-oriented culture.	Routine monitoring of customers' views. Every opportunity taken to involve users in designing service at personal level.

Medium	Appreciable number of individual projects, still not well coordinated but using common approaches to problem-solving etc. Some part-time support from untrained quality facilitators for some groups.	Beginning to see shift from perception of importance of internal/external customer focus to empowerment and difference between absolute resource constraints and making more effective use of resources.	A critical mass, say 30–40% are involved in some way in collecting data on own and work group's performance. Users are built in, in limited way, in some processes. Tendency still to be reactive and problem-oriented.	Some information going out to customers and occasional surveys undertaken. Nearly all *post hoc.*
Low	One or two quality initiatives driven by committed individuals, but uncoordinated. Little/no management support. Complaints about management criticizing staff rather than supporting them are common.	Little/no sense of the importance of internal customers but increasing commitment to external customer focus. Defensive barriers between staff in different departments. Professional/technical definitions of quality hold sway.	Little involvement of staff beyond QIGs or standard-setting groups. Data collection is problem-oriented and dominated by static models of standard-setting and annual audits. Rarely lead to increasing standards.	Feedback from customers is tapped sporadically and on personal basis only. No systematic monitoring or evaluation.

References

Atkinson, P. E. (1990) Creating culture change – the key to successful total quality management, *TQM Magazine*, IFS Ltd, Bedford.

Audit Commission (1992) *Minding the Quality: A Consultation Document on the Role of the Audit Commission in Quality Assurance and Health Care.* Audit Commission, London.

Becher, T. and Kogan, M. (1992) *Process and Structure in Higher Education.* Routledge, London.

Bell, L., Brown, R. and Morris, B. (1993) Auditing Health and Community Services from a New Perspective in *Quality and its Applications.* University of Newcastle on Tyne.

Bertram, D. (1993) *The Role of Junior and Middle Level Management in TQM*, TQM Practitioner Series. Technical Communications (Publishing) Ltd., Letchworth.

Berwick, D., Enthoven, A. and Bunker, J. (1992a) 'Quality management in the NHS: the doctor's role – I', *British Medical Journal*, vol. 304, pp. 235–9.

Berwick, D., Enthoven, A. and Bunker, J. (1992b) 'Quality management in the NHS: the doctor's role – II', *British Medical Journal*, vol. 304, pp. 304–8.

Bitner, M. (1991) 'The evolution of the services marketing mix and its relationship to service quality' in S. W. Brown, E. Gummesson, B. Edvardsson and B. Gustavsson (eds), *Service Quality – Multidisciplinary and Multinational Perspectives.* Lexington Books, Lexington, MA.

Braybrooke, D. and Lindblom, C. (1963) *A Strategy of Decision.* Collier Macmillan, London.

Brown, S. W., Gummesson, E., Edvardsson, B. and Gustavsson, B. (eds) (1991) *Service Quality – Multidisciplinary and Multinational Perspectives.* Lexington Books, Lexington, MA.

Burns, T. (1977) *The BBC: Public Institution and Private World.* Macmillan, London.

Burns, T. (1981) 'Rediscovering organisational aspects of collaboration and managerialism in hospital organisations', unpublished. Referred to in Hunter (1983).

Buxton, M., Packwood, T. and Keen, J. (1991) *Resource Management: Final Report of the Brunel University Evaluation of Resource Management*. Brunel University, Uxbridge.

Carswell, L. and McAlister, D. (1991) 'Is resource management simply gloss without a quality undercoat? A hospital perspective', paper presented to the Study Group on Productivity and Quality in the Public Sector, European Group for Public Administration, 29 August–21 September 1991.

Chase, R. and Bowen, D. (1991) 'Service quality and the service delivery system – a diagnostic framework' in S. W. Brown, E. Gummesson, B. Edwardsson and B. Gustavesson (eds), *Service Quality – Multidisciplinary and Multinational Perspectives*. Lexington Books, Lexington, MA.

Chin, R. and Benn, K. (1969) 'The roots of planned change' in W. Bennis, K. Benn and R. Chin, *The Planning of Change* (2nd edn). Holt, Reinhart and Winston, New York.

Crosby, P. B. (1979) *Quality is Free*. McGraw-Hill, New York.

Crosby, P. B. (1988) *The Eternally Successful Organization*. McGraw-Hill, New York.

Czepiel, J., Solomon, M. and Surprenant, C. (1985) The *Service Encounter*, Lexington Books, Lexington, Massachusetts.

Dalley, G. and Carr-Hill, R. (1991) *Pathways to Quality, A Study of Quality Management Initiatives in the NHS. A Guide for Managers*, Quality Management Initiatives No. 2, Centre for Health Economics, University of York.

Deming, W. (1986) *Out of the Crisis*. Massachusetts Institute of Technology, Cambridge, MA.

Department of Health (1989) *Medical Audit – Working Paper No. 6. Working for Patients*. HMSO, London.

Department of Health (1992) *Local Voices, The Views of Local People in Purchasing for Health*, NHS Management Executive, Leeds.

Department of Health (1993a) *Monitoring Made Easy*. Patient's Charter Unit, Health Publications, Lancs.

Department of Health (1993b) *The Quality Journey: A Guide to Total Quality Management in the NHS*. NHS Management Executive, Leeds.

Donabedian, A. (1980) *The Definition of Quality and Approaches to its Management, Vol. 1: Explorations in Quality Assessment and Monitoring*. Health Administration Press, Ann Arbor, MI.

Donabedian, A. (1982) *The Criteria and Standards of Quality, Vol. 2: Explorations in Quality Assessment and Monitoring*. Health Administration Press, Ann Arbor, MI.

Donabedian, A. (1988) 'The quality of care – how can it be assessed?', *Journal of the American Medical Association*, vol. 260, no. 12, pp. 1743–8.

Edvardsson, B. and Gustavsson, B. (1991) 'Quality in services and quality in service organisations – a model for quality assessment' in S. W. Brown, E. Gummesson, B. Edvardsson and B. Gustavsson (eds), *Service Quality – Multidisciplinary and Multinational Perspectives*. Lexington Books, Lexington, MA.

Edvardsson, B., Thomasson, B. and Øvretveit, J. (1994) *Quality of Service*. McGraw-Hill, Maidenhead.

Elmore, R. (1982) 'Backward mapping: implementation research and policy decisions' in W. Williams (ed.), *Studying Implementation: Methodological and Administrative Issues*. Chatham House Publishers, Chatham, NJ.

Evans, K. and Corrigan, P. (1990) 'Standard setting: an introduction to differing approaches', *Nursing Practice*, vol. 4, no. 3, pp. 16–19.

Gaster, L. (1991) 'Quality and decentralisation: are they connected?', *Policy and Politics*, vol. 19, no. 4.

Griffiths, R. (1983) *NHS Management Enquiry: Report*. Department of Health and Social Services, London.

Gronroos, C. (1984) 'A service quality model and its marketing implications', *European Journal of Marketing*, vol. 18, no. 4.

Hammer, M. and Champy, J. (1993) *Reengineering the Corporation – A Manifesto for Business Revolution*. Nicholas Brealey Publishing, London.

Harrison, S., Hunter, D., Marnoch, G. and Pollitt, C. (1989) *The Impact of General Management in the National Health Service*. The Open University and Nuffield Institute for Health Service Studies, Milton Keynes.

Harvey, L., Burrows, A. and Green, D. (1993) *Criteria of Quality*. Quality in Higher Education Project, University of Central England, Birmingham.

Henkel, M. (1992) *Government, Evaluation and Change*. Jessica Kingsley Publishers, London.

Hirschman, A. (1970) *Exit, Voice and Loyalty: Responses to Decline in Firms, Organizations and States*. Harvard University Press, Cambridge, MA.

Hoggett, P. (1991) 'A new management in the public sector?', *Policy and Politics*, vol. 19, no. 4.

Hunter, D. (1983) 'Centre–periphery relations in the NHS: facilitators or inhibitors of innovation' in K. Young (ed.), *National Interests and Local Government*. Heinemann Educational Books, London.

Ishikawa, K. (1985) *What is Total Quality Control? The Japanese Way*. Prentice Hall, Englewood Cliffs, NJ.

Jaques, E. (1976) *A General Theory of Bureaucracy*. Heinemann Educational Books, Portsmouth, NH.

Jaques, E. (1989) *Requisite Organisation: The CEO's Guide to Creative Structure and Leadership*. Cason Hall and Co., Arlington, Virginia, USA.

Joss, R. (1994a) 'Converging implementation strategies in commercial TQM initiatives: implications for the NHS', *International Journal of Health Care Quality Assurance*, vol. 7, no. 2.

Joss, R. (1994b) 'What makes for successful TQM in the NHS?', *International Journal of Health Care Quality Assurance*, vol. 7, no. 7.

Joss, R., Kogan, M. and Henkel, M. (1992) *Third Interim Report to the Department of Health, October 1992*. Centre for the Evaluation of Public Policy and Practice, Brunel, The University of West London, Uxbridge.

Joss, R., Kogan, M. and Henkel, M. (1991) *First Interim Report to the Department of Health, November 1991*. Centre for the Evaluation of Public Policy and Practice, Brunel University, Uxbridge.

Joss, R., Kogan, M. and Henkel, M. (1994) *Total Quality Management in the National Health Service: Final Report of an Evaluation to the Department of Health*. Centre for the Evaluation of Public Policy and Practice, Brunel University, Uxbridge.

Joss, R. (1995) 'A case study on the cost of quality in an NHS hospital' in G. Bouckaert and C. Pollitt (eds), *Quality Improvement in European Public Services: Concepts, Cases and Commentary*. Sage, London.

Juran, J. (1988) *Juran on Planning for Quality*. The Free Press, New York.

Kackar, R. N. (1985) 'Off-line quality control parameter design and the Taguchi method', *Journal of Quality Technology*, vol. 17, pp. 176–88.

Klaus, P. (1985) 'Quality epiphenomenon: the conceptual understanding of quality in face to face service encounters', in J. Czepiel, M. Solomon, and C. Surprenant (eds), *The Service Encounter*. Lexington Books, Lexington, MA.

Koch, H. (1993) Papers presented at 1993 ICM Conference on TQM in the NHS, London.

Kogan, M., Cang, S., Dixon, M. and Tolliday, H. (1971) *Working Relationships Within the British Hospital Service*. Bookstall Publications, London.

Kogan, M., Redfern, S., Kober, A., Norman, I., Packwood, T. and Robinson, S. (1995a) *Clinical Audit in Four Health Professions*. Joint Report by the Centre for the Evaluation of Public Policy and Practice and the Nursing Research Unit, King's College, London University.

Kogan, M., Redfern, S., Kober, A., Norman, I., Packwood, T. and Robinson, S. (1995b) *Making Use Of Clinical Audit*. Open University Press, Buckingham.

Lewin, K. (1952), *Field Theory in Social Science: Selected Theoretical Papers*. Tavistock Publications, London.

Macdonald, I., Macdonald, R. and Stewart, K. (1989) 'Leadership: a new direction', *British Army Review*, December.

Macdonald, J. (1993) *TQM: Does it always Work?*. TQM Practitioners Series, Technical Communications (Publishing) Ltd., Letchworth.

Macdonald, J. and Piggott, J. (1990) *Global Quality – The New Management Culture*. Mercury Books, London.

Maxwell, R. (1984) 'Quality assessment in Health', *British Medical Journal*, vol. 288, pp. 1470–72.

Merrifield, A. (1990a) Lead article, *NHS Management Executive News*, no. 37, September, pp. 1–2.

Merrifield, A. (1990b) 'The NHS and its consumers', opening address to the Conference on Total Quality Management in the NHS, Birmingham, November.

Nader, R. (1965) *Unsafe at any Speed: The Designed-in Dangers of the American Automobile*. Grossman, New York.

Neave, G. (1988) 'On the cultivation of quality, efficiency and enterprise: an overview of recent trends in higher education in Europe, 1986–1988', *European Journal of Education*, vol. 23, nos 1–2.

Neave, H. (1990) *The Deming Dimension*. SPC Press Inc., Knoxville, TN.

Neuhauser, P. (1988) *Tribal Warfare in Organizations*. Balinger, Cambridge, MA.

Oakland, J. S. (1989) *Total Quality Management*. Heinemann, Oxford.

Øvretveit, J. (1990) 'What is quality in health services?', *Health Services Management*, vol. 86, no. 3, pp. 132–3.

Øvretveit, J. (1992) *Health Service Quality: An Introduction to Quality Methods for Health Services*. Blackwell Scientific Publications, Oxford.

Parasuraman, A., Zeithaml, V. and Berry, L. (1985) 'A conceptual model of service quality and its implications for future research', *Journal of Marketing*, vol. 49, pp. 41–50.

Peters, T. (1989) *Thriving on Chaos – Handbook for a Management Revolution*. Pan Books, London.

Pfeffer, N. and Coote, A. (1991) *Is Quality Good for You? – A Critical Review of Quality Assurance in Welfare Services*. Institute for Public Policy Research, London.

Pollitt, C. (1990) 'Doing business in the temple? Managers and quality assurance in the public services', *Public Administration*, vol. 68, no. 4, pp. 435–52.

Rein, M. (1983) 'Implementation: a theoretical perspective' in *Policy to Practice*. Macmillan Press, New York.

Rosander, A. (1989) *The Quest for Quality in Services.* Quality Press, American Society for Quality Control, Milwaukee, WI.

Royal College of Nursing (1991) *Total Quality Management – A Framework for Quality Care.* Royal College of Nursing of the United Kingdom, NHS General Managers Forum, London.

Schön, D. (1983) *The Reflective Practitioner: How Professionals Think in Action.* Temple Smith, London.

Scriven, M. (1967) 'The methodology of evaluation' in *Perspectives of Curriculum Evaluation*, AERA Monograph No. 1. Rand McNally, Chicago.

Shewhart, W. A. (1931) *Economic Control of Quality of Manufactured Product.* Van Nostrand, New York.

Shostack, L. (1987) 'Service positioning through structural change', *Journal of Marketing*, vol. 51, pp. 34–43.

Sketris, I. (1988) *Health Service Accreditation – An International Overview.* King's Fund Centre.

Steffen, G. (1988) 'Quality medical care – a definition', *Journal of the American Medical Association*, vol. 260, no. 1.

Suchman, E. (1967) *Evaluative Research, Principles and Practice in Public Service and Social Action Programs.* Russell Sage Foundation, New York.

Thompson, D. (1992) *The Changing Face of the National Health Service in the 1990s* (ed. P. Spurgeon). Health Services Management Centre, Longman, Harlow.

TQM Magazine (1991) *Cross Functional Teams and Teamwork*, February 1991, IFS Publications, Bedford, UK

Tuckman, A. and Blackburn, D. (1991) 'Fitness for purpose: Total Quality Management in the health service', paper presented at the BSA Annual Conference, Manchester, March.

Waldegrave, W. (1991) 'Developing the purchasing role', in *NHS Management Executive News*, no. 45, May, p. 5.

Williamson, J. (1991) 'Providing quality care', *Health Services Management*, vol. 87, no. 1, pp. 18–23.

Wolman, H. (1984) 'The determinants of program success and failure', *Journal of Public Policy*, vol. 1, no. 4, pp. 433–64.

Woodward, J. (1965) *Industrial Theory and Practice.* Oxford University Press, Oxford.

Index

PURCHASING FOR HEALTH
A MULTIDISCIPLINARY INTRODUCTION TO THE THEORY AND PRACTICE OF HEALTH PURCHASING

John Øvretveit

Health purchasing has grown in prominence as a result of health reform in Europe and the USA to become one of the world's biggest industries. People's health increasingly depends on the skills and abilities of health purchasing managers, yet little is known about the subject. Ordinary people are becoming aware of the sums spent in their name by 'faceless bureaucrats', and cannot see what value health purchasers add. Although health purchasing is more than paying bills and contracting services, there is uncertainty about the purpose and future role of purchasing organizations in different health systems.

This first book on the subject views health purchasing – both public and private – as a service industry. It argues that, to survive, purchasers have to be more than agents of cost control and must win public support by shaping technological and service changes to uphold our rights and interests. Purchasers need to use service management methods and organization to improve their services to ordinary people.

This book contributes to the theory and practice of the new management discipline of health purchasing, and to an understanding of health purchasing organizations, both public and private. It examines the purpose and methods of health purchasing as a service industry in a rapidly changing and unique type of market. Although concentrating on public health purchasing in the British National Health Service, the book does so in a way which allows comparisons to be made with purchasing in other countries. It presents practical approaches, concepts, and models which have helped purchasing managers and governing board members to tackle key issues. It draws on experience from a variety of sources including a development programme for seven integrated NHS purchasing agencies and the author's research into health reforms in Europe and the USA.

Contents
Purchasing for health – Purchasing and 'market reform' – Health commissioning: purpose and work – 'Decentralized' or 'locality' purchasing – Justifiable purchasing: rationing, priorities, effectiveness and outcome – Contracting and contracts – Quality in purchasing – Collaboration with local authorities – Developing primary and community health services – Purchasing primary health care and the role of the FHSA – Integrating primary and secondary health purchasing – Purchasing agency organization – The future for health purchasing: financing, competition and values – References – Bibliography – Index.

368pp   0 335 19332 3 (Paperback)   0 335 19333 1 (Hardback)